MOSBY'S

TOUR GUIDE

TO NURSING SCHOOL

In Collaboration with

NSNA

NATIONAL STUDENT NURSES' ASSOCIATION

MOSBY'S

TOUR GUIDE

TO NURSING SCHOOL

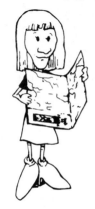

A STUDENT'S ROAD SURVIVAL KIT

THIRD EDITION

Melodie Chenevert, R.N., B.S.N., M.N., M.A.
Pro-Nurse
Gaithersburg, MD

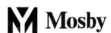 Mosby

A *Harcourt Health Sciences Company*
St. Louis Philadelphia London Sydney Toronto

Printed in the United States of America

Mosby, Inc.
11830 Westline industrial drive
St. Louis, Missouri 63146

Library of Congress Cataloging-in-Publication Data
Chenevert, Melodie
    Mosby's tour guide to nursing school : a student's road survival
kit / Melodie Chenevert.—3rd ed.
        p.   cm.
    "In collaboration with NSNA, National Student Nurses'
Association"—P. [1] of cover.
    Includes bibliographical references and index.
    ISBN 0–8151–1539–3
    1. Nursing students.   2. Nursing schools.   3. Nursing—Vocational
guidance.   4. Success.   I. National Student Nurses' Association
(U.S.)   II. Title.   III. Title: Tour guide to nursing school.
    [DNLM: 1. Schools, Nursing—popular works.   2. Education, Nursing
—popular works.   WY 19 C518m 1995]
RT73.C49   1995
610.73'071'1—dc20
DNLM/DLC
                                                                    94-32030

00 01 02 / 9 8 7 6 5 4

Note to Students

Any nursing student will tell you that going to nursing school entails a lot more than just going to classes. Unlike many majors, nursing school seems to encompass your whole life. Whether it's because of the complexity of the materials, long clinical hours, short periods of sleep or all of a sudden being in such close proximity to so many other students who are also having to adjust to their own set of changes—a nursing student's life will never be the same.

Mosby's Tour Guide To Nursing School offers practical and often comical insight into situations that nursing students face on a daily basis. It offers practical suggestions to beginning students as well as those about to graduate. While reading this book I laughed and was comforted when I often thought of myself in many of the situations described by Melodie Chenevert.

The National Student Nurses' Association (NSNA) is pleased to have the opportunity to participate in this publication. NSNA is committed to preparing nursing students for the challenges that will face them as students and as professionals—and *Mosby's Tour Guide to Nursing School* will serve as a great resource.

Take the time to read, laugh, and learn. Remember, one day we will look back on our experiences in nursing school with a chuckle, a sigh, and the satisfaction of having accomplished our goal.

Bill Lightfoot
NSNA President

Foreword

I am always delighted to have the opportunity to write the foreword for *Mosby's Tour Guide to Nursing School: A Student's Road Survival Kit*. The candor and humor of this edition is noteworthy. Typical academic, social and personal experiences portrayed by the author are very true to life, in spite of their humor. These are experiences that nursing students do, in fact, encounter. Melodie Chenevert does a fine job of describing ways in which nursing students can overcome the many difficulties they are likely to encounter during their education. Stressful situations that can and do arise during nursing school are dealt with by providing students with sound advice for coping.

This book is fast and easy reading. The adage that "Many a truth is said in jest" is demonstrated by this work. The concerns of students described in the book are true to life, and encountered every day. These issues are timeless. I continue to hear of them from students across the country.

Mosby's Tour Guide to Nursing School: A Student's Road Survival Kit is a useful tool for students. I believe it should be part of every nursing student's personal library. It provides helpful hints in a light, humorous fashion that makes the book easy to use. It's refreshing, as one reads, to pause and smile at oneself. There are many lessons to be learned from this publication.

I am delighted that the National Student Nurses' Association has played a small role in the production of this work.

Robert V. Piemonte, EdD, RN, CAE, FAAN
Executive Director
National Student Nurses' Association, Inc.

Preface

In Houston at a city-wide extravaganza honoring graduating nursing students, a young man glanced at my name tag. "You!" he exclaimed. "You're the person who wrote that book! You're the person who got me through nursing school!" He grabbed me and gave me a big hug.

It was a wonderful moment. I have never been more proud of being the author of *Mosby's Tour Guide to Nursing School*. It's a book that has helped lots of people get through nursing school and it can help you too.

You are holding the third edition. Everything has been updated. One outstanding feature of this survival guide is that it tackles the challenges faced by "mature" students. Nursing educators used to call anyone over 20 and other than female a "nontraditional" student. Today female students under 20 are the exception, not the rule. Although typical nursing students are still overwhelmingly female, they are not as young as they used to be. They're older and wiser and much more encumbered. They bring a lot of baggage—obligations, responsibilities, commitments, constraints, and conflicts—all of which make being a successful student much more challenging.

Although this book is primarily designed for the "first-time travelers," nurses returning for advanced degrees and experienced students from other fields making a career switch into nursing have reported the strategies and suggestions in the *Tour Guide* most helpful.

So grab a copy of this book and come on along. You are about to embark on a great journey. Destination: NURSING. It's a rough trip but worth every mile.

Most travelers on this route have a lot in common. Most of us are practical idealists. You know—the sort of people who want to save the human race but who also know the value of a regular paycheck.

As a practical idealist myself, I know it's not easy keeping your feet on the ground while your head's in the clouds. Nursing is one of the few professions that enables you to make such a long stretch.

Nursing is practically ideal. You will not only earn a good living, you will help others in the process. You will have the knowledge and skills to convert your good intentions into good actions. Although you will not be able to save the whole planet, occasionally you will save one of its occupants. That will be enough. And you will be paid for your services, although perhaps not as much as your skill will deserve.

Nursing school can make you wise beyond your years, but it sometimes also makes you old before your time. This tour guide/survival kit will help you achieve more in nursing school with less wear and tear on your body, mind, and spirit.

Too many "sky's-the-limit" students trip over their own shoelaces. So this book is designed to make sure you don't lose your footing or your ideals. Its down-to-earth tips can help make an average student good and a good student great.

Here's the information you need on everything from boosting your test scores to boosting your self-esteem, from conducting a study group to overcoming procrastination, from choosing electives to improving term papers to avoiding collisions between your personal and professional lives. Plus you will find candid comments, examples, and ideas from other nursing students.

From the beginning this book has been a collaborative effort. Not only has it involved Mosby, the National Student Nurses' Association, and me, it reflects input from countless students and nurses throughout the United States and Canada.

There is only one person who can make this book any better: YOU! Your input can make sure this tour guide/survival kit keeps doing the job it was designed to do—help nursing students survive and even thrive.

If you would like to make a suggestion, share an experience, give a recommendation, or pass along a hot tip, write to me. I promise to respond.

Bon voyage!

Melodie Chenevert
c/o Nursing Division, Mosby–Year Book, Inc.
11830 Westline Industrial Drive
St. Louis, MO 63146

Contents

I THE STARTING LINEUP   3

If you've been admitted to a school of nursing, you can do anything! Cooperation, not competition, will bring success.

2 IS THIS TRIP REALLY NECESSARY?   5

Determining whether you have what it takes to be a nurse. Diverse demands on a working nurse.

3 DESTINATION: REGISTERED NURSE   II

Tangible and intangible rewards of nursing.

4 HOW LONG WILL THIS TRIP TAKE?   17

Three preparatory paths to nursing. Career aspirations and financial and time considerations determine the length of education.

5 HOW MUCH WILL THIS TRIP COST?   23

Calculating and defraying expenses. Being a smart consumer and getting your money's worth.

6 RULES OF THE ROAD 29

Don't fight the system—work with it. Know your school's rules and follow them to the letter. Collisions between personal freedoms and professional responsibilities.

7 SLOWER TRAFFIC KEEP RIGHT 33

Survival tips from students to students: take care of yourself, take care of each other, take one day at a time, and take care of business.

8 DRIVING INSTRUCTORS 37

The importance of knowing faculty members thoroughly and understanding the many roles they play.

9 MORE MILES PER GALLON 43

Time management from A to Z.

10 DETOURS 53

Turning wishes into goals and goals into accomplishments. Issues for the student who must work while going to school.

11 YOU CAN'T GET THERE FROM HERE 59

Problem solving and assertiveness skills.

12 DRIVE-UP TELLER 65

Making the best use of your memory bank: listening and learning; reading and remembering.

13 TOLLBOOTH 75

Test-taking skills designed to boost your grades.

14 TOTALED 85

Dealing with failure: major or minor.

15 HOW TO JUMP-START YOUR BATTERY 91

Procrastination and motivation.

16 10-4, GOOD BUDDY 97

How to form and conduct study groups. Supporting each other.

17 PREVENTIVE MAINTENANCE   105

The importance of taking care of yourself.

18 SCENIC ROUTES   109

Choosing electives.

19 ALTERNATE ROUTES   113

Diversity within the nursing profession. Increasing tolerance and flexibility. How to keep judgmental attitudes from interfering with professional performance.

20 BUSINESS ROUTES   117

Improving oral and written reports.

21 IN THE DRIVER'S SEAT   125

Taking full responsibility for your actions.

22 SHIFTING GEARS   127

Difficulties of being a spouse/parent/student; challenges of returning to school after a long absence; making the transition from person to professional.

23 MOVING VIOLATIONS   139

Making the most of the nursing skills lab; getting adequate experience in the clinical setting.

24 DEFENSIVE DRIVING   145

Rights and responsibilities. Conforming to the letter or the spirit of the law. Paperwork.

25 STREET SMART   159

Surviving on tough turf. The importance of first impressions and body language.

26 LIFE IN THE FAST LANE   165

Last-minute suggestions from senior students.

27 ARE WE THERE YET?   169

Transition from experienced student to inexperienced professional. But if you have gotten this far, you can do anything!

Appendixes

A   RESOURCES FOR NCLEX REVIEW   171

B   GRIEVANCE PROCEDURE GUIDELINES   177

C   COMMON PREFIXES AND SUFFIXES USED IN
    NURSING   183

D   SOURCES OF SCHOLARSHIPS AND
    LOANS   189

E   QUESTIONS AND ANSWERS ON THE
    COMPUTERIZED NCLEX-RN EXAM   193

F   U.S. STATE AND TERRITORIAL BOARDS OF
    NURSING   197

G   U.S. AND CANADIAN NURSING
    ORGANIZATIONS   201

H   SPECIALIZED NURSING ORGANIZATIONS IN
    THE UNITED STATES AND CANADA   205

MOSBY'S

TOUR GUIDE

TO NURSING SCHOOL

Dedicated to the future nurse
and
the future of nursing . . .
they are one and the same

"It is a rough road that leads
to the heights of greatness."

SENECA

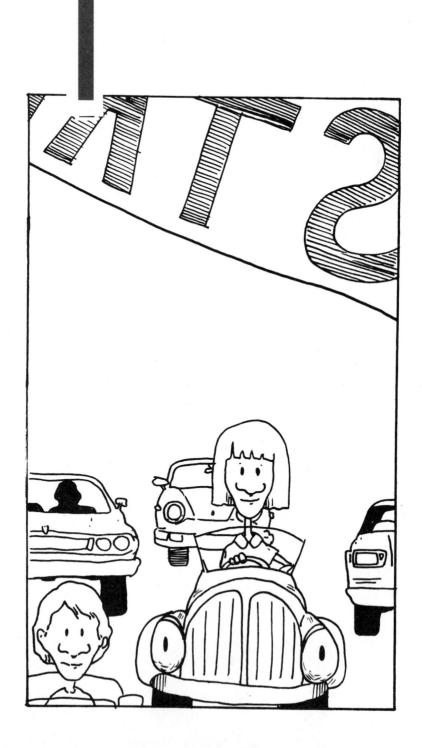

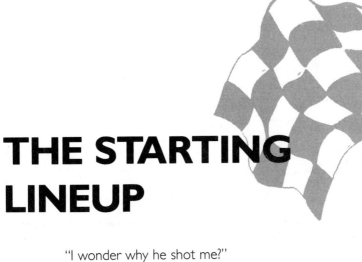

THE STARTING LINEUP

"I wonder why he shot me?"
—Huey Long

The first thing many students do is size up the competition. They think of getting an education as a fiercely competitive race. They jockey for first position as though only one student will be allowed to graduate.

Whether or not you're this competitive, it's only human to look at your classmates and wonder about your comparative status. You may even begin to wonder whether the faculty knew what they were doing when they admitted you. After all, how can they expect you to compete with a fellow who served as a medic in Vietnam, a woman who is old enough to be your mother, a high school valedictorian, and a person who holds a bachelor's degree in psychology?

Relax. You are not expected to *compete* with other students. You are expected to *cooperate* with them.

Instead of a race, think of this educational venture as a caravan about to undertake a long journey. The ultimate goal is to get everyone in your class to the final destination. It is cooperation, not competition, that will bring you success.

Everyone in your class has an excellent chance to graduate because everyone here is already a winner. All have won a place at the starting gate. Considering the rigors of the admission process, getting here was no small accomplishment. If you have managed to get admitted to a school of nursing, YOU CAN DO ANYTHING!

So start your engines. We're off and running.

3

2

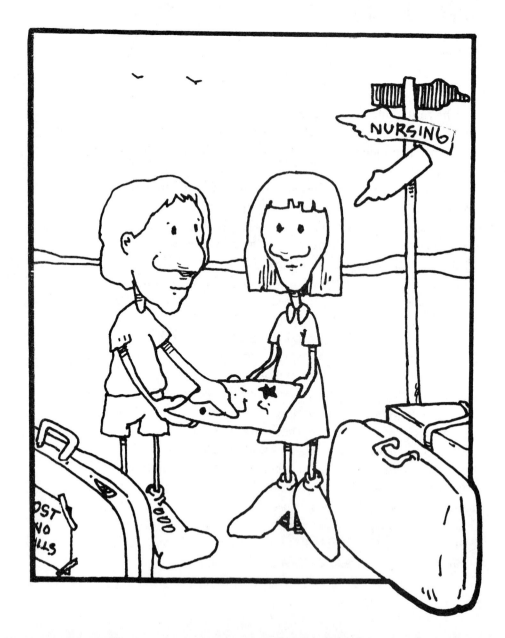

IS THIS TRIP REALLY NECESSARY?

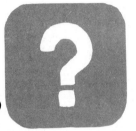

"I shall be telling this with a sigh
Somewhere ages and ages hence:
Two roads diverged in a wood,
and I—I took the one less traveled by,
And that has made all the difference."
—Robert Frost,
The Road Not Taken

Before you begin this long journey, double-check to make sure you know where you are going and what you will find when you get there. If you want to work as a nurse, you are on the right road. If you actually want to work as an airline flight attendant or a health care administrator, you are on the wrong road or, at least, the *long* road. Don't think of nursing education as a "good background" or a "springboard" to another job or profession.

While men grow up expecting to work a lifetime, women grow up expecting to work part time. Yet Department of Labor statistics indicate that the average woman can expect to marry, have two children, and work full time for 30 to 40 years! Do not underestimate the importance of the work you select.

People who choose nursing usually have other interests besides just making a living. They are looking for a way of life that is compatible with their humanitarian instincts.

Having a relative or a friend with a severe handicap or health problem can be a real source of inspiration. It can also be a real source of guilt. Sometimes people who venture into nursing are on guilt trips. They are trying to make up for things that happened in the past.

WHAT IT IS, AND WHAT IT ISN'T

If you think nursing is an insurance policy—something nice to "fall back on" in case you are forced to work at some point in the future—think again. Rapid developments in science and technology make it difficult even for working nurses to keep their skills current.

Nurses who drop out of the profession for a few years have been finding it increasingly difficult, and often impossible, to re-enter. The once-a-nurse-always-a-nurse guarantee may have expired. For example, an Iowa nurse who had been out of the profession for 10 years decided to return to nursing. At every interview she was told that first choice in hiring went to employed nurses seeking transfers, second choice went to new graduates, and third choice went to former nurses who had completed a refresher course. The Catch-22 was that there were no refresher courses being offered in Iowa at that time.

If you think nursing is the road to perpetual job security, think again. For more than 40 years (1942 to the mid-1980s), that was essentially true because the demand for nurses exceeded the supply. By 1984, however, astonished nurses in many parts of the United States suddenly faced layoffs and a very tight job market.

Although analysts saw this "surplus" of nurses as an artificial glitch and predicted the shortage would soon reappear, the damage was already done. Potential nursing students turned away from the profession in droves. In 1986 schools of nursing reported drops in enrollment of *up to 50 percent.*

That bad news proved to be good news for nurses and nursing students. As the economy recovered, the demand for nurses skyrocketed. Funding for education increased. Salaries shot up dramatically. Hospitals went to great lengths to attract and keep good nurses.

The nurse shortage made national headlines. Schools of nurses were filled to overflowing. In 1993, for every student admitted to a school of nursing, two students had to be turned away.

But by then the nation's economy was in serious trouble. The early 1990s looked just like the early 1980s. The nurse shortage? What nurse shortage? Hospitals were merging, downsizing, closing. Suddenly experienced nurses flooded the market. In many areas of the country, new graduates were hard pressed to find entry-level positions.

Boom. Bust. Boom. Bust.

Health care reform is inevitable, but what that reform will actually entail is anyone's guess. It promises to be an exciting time for nurses.

Today two-thirds of all nurses work in hospitals. By the year 2000, however, projections are that the number of hospital beds will be cut in half. That doesn't mean people won't need care. It means they will need care in other settings— the home, the school, the clinic, the community. You will hear a lot about "advanced practice nurses." These will be nurses with graduate degrees who are equipped to provide that sort of primary care.

So before you follow the yellow brick road to nursing, you should be sure to separate fact from fantasy. For example, if you think a nurse's primary function is to assist the doctor, you have been watching too much television. In real life nurses spend very little time working alongside doctors. Nurses usually work alone.

WHAT DO NURSES DO ALL DAY?

Nursing is not a do-as-you-are-told job. It is a profession that demands the ability to interview, observe, analyze, detect, develop, write, teach, interpret, counsel, coordinate, collaborate, insert, inject, dispense, change, document, count, order, improvise, supervise, create, give, and take.

In one day you may be called on to do such diverse tasks as interview patients, document progress, develop care plans, write discharge summaries, teach self-care, interpret laboratory findings, insert tubes, check monitors, maintain life-support machinery, counsel grief-stricken families, collaborate with other health-care professionals, analyze problems, assess potentials, irrigate wounds, change dressings, collect specimens, coordinate care during birth or death, dispense medications, take temperatures, and give hope.

Much of a nurse's time is spent in direct patient care. Most nurses wish it could be more. Unfortunately, nurses are also saddled with lots of other tasks, such as transcribing doctors' orders, counting narcotics, ordering supplies, directing traffic, enforcing policies, maintaining schedules, answering telephones, delivering dinner trays, cleaning utility rooms, fetching equipment, running errands, and mopping up messes.

The general-duty, all-purpose, industrial-strength registered nurse must be ready, willing, and able to deliver everything from mail to babies. Obviously it takes much more than a nice personality, a ready smile, and good intentions to make a good nurse. Yet every year parents, friends, neighbors, and even high school counselors encourage people with more fluff than substance to take up nursing.

Are you fluff or substance? To find out, take this quiz:

DO YOU HAVE ...

1. A strong background in math and science?   □ Yes   □ No

2. Good hand-eye coordination?   □ Yes   □ No

3. Lots of common sense?   □ Yes   □ No

4. The ability to stay calm in emergencies?   □ Yes   □ No

5. Excellent communication skills?   □ Yes   □ No

6. A sound body?   □ Yes   □ No

7. A stable mind?   □ Yes   □ No

8. An above-average intellect?   □ Yes   □ No

9. An affinity for machines and computers? ☐ Yes ☐ No

10. A compassionate heart? ☐ Yes ☐ No

11. Teaching abilities? ☐ Yes ☐ No

12. Leadership qualities? ☐ Yes ☐ No

13. Patience, tolerance, flexibility, persistence? ☐ Yes ☐ No

14. A strong ego? ☐ Yes ☐ No

15. An affinity for problem solving? ☐ Yes ☐ No

16. Confidence in your decision-making abilities? ☐ Yes ☐ No

17. Good organizational skills? ☐ Yes ☐ No

18. Reliable powers of observation? ☐ Yes ☐ No

19. The ability to see the best in people in the worst of times? ☐ Yes ☐ No

20. No objection to working on Christmas? ☐ Yes ☐ No

FILL IN ONE BLOCK FOR EVERY "YES" ANSWER

FLUFF   SUBSTANCE

☐ ☐ ☐ ☐ ☐ ☐ ☐ ☐ ☐ ☐ ☐ ☐ ☐ ☐ ☐ ☐ ☐ ☐ ☐ ☐

If you have all of the above qualities, skip nursing and go directly to sainthood. You are not only too good for nursing, you are too good to be true. But the more of these attributes you have, the more likely you are to make a success of nursing—and the more likely nursing is to make a success of you.

3

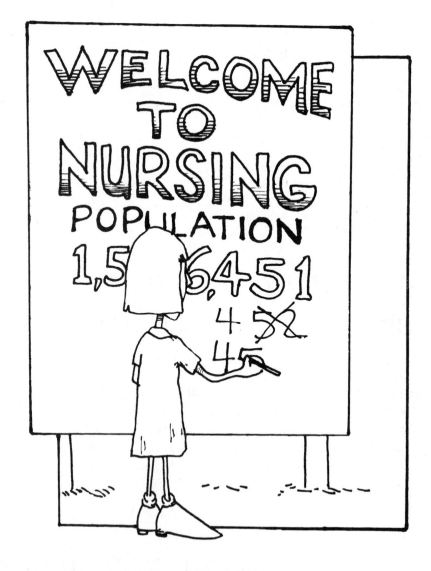

DESTINATION: REGISTERED NURSE

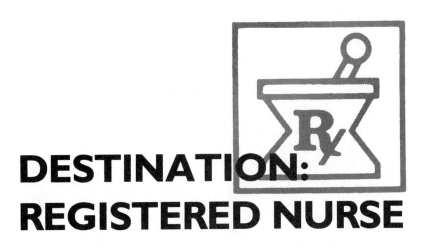

"If I can throw any obscurity on the
subject please let me know."
—James Joyce

Welcome to nursing! The most exasperating career ever
invented. It is also the most fulfilling. I can guarantee you intangible rewards that can rarely be matched by any other
profession. I can also guarantee that as a nurse:

You will never be bored.

You will always be frustrated.

You will be surrounded by challenges—so much to do and
    so little time.

You will carry immense responsibility with very little au-
    thority.

You will step into people's lives, and you will make a dif-
    ference.

Some will bless you. Some will curse you.

You will see people at their worst—and at their best. You will never cease to be amazed at people's capacity for love, courage, and endurance.

You will see life begin and end.

You will experience resounding triumphs and devastating failures.

You will cry a lot.

You will laugh a lot.

You will know what it is to be human and to be humane.

What I cannot guarantee are tangible rewards as rich as the intangible ones. Nursing is fraught with all the problems facing any job category that is manned overwhelmingly by women.

What tangible rewards can you expect from nursing? The quickest way to assess your future earning potential is to look at the most current career-opportunity guides published annually by nursing journal companies. Hospitals spend big bucks advertising in these guides, hoping to entice nurses to come work for them.

NURSING CAREER GUIDE DECODER KIT

As you investigate salaries, it may appear that there are some significant variations around the country. However, if you adjust those salaries in terms of cost of living, the differences effectively evaporate. For example, it costs twice as much to live half as well in New York City as it does in rural Georgia.

You will also notice that a mere $2000 may separate starting salaries for new graduates from starting salaries for experienced nurses. In addition, you should know that the vast majority of hospitals make no monetary distinction between nurses who have a bachelor's degree and those who do not.

Hospitals that do reward higher education may pay as little as $500 per year for a bachelor's degree and $1000 for a master's degree.

At the height of the last nurse shortage, these were some of the perquisites hospitals were proud to offer:

"Relocation allowance"

"37.5-hour work week"

"12 holidays per year"

"4 weeks of vacation"

"Half of all weekends off"

"Tuition reimbursement for senior year"

"$500 differential for BSN"

"NO SHIFT ROTATION"

"Uniform allowance"

"Weekend bonus of 25%"

"Free parking"

"Dental insurance"

"Discounts on prescription drugs"

"Tax-sheltered annuities"

"Evening/night differentials"
(Ranging from less than $1500 to more than $7500 per year)

Read between the lines. This is the good stuff. These hospitals are boasting. That means a lot of hospitals offer less: less vacation, fewer holidays, no tuition reimbursement, no uniform allowance, no bonuses for weekend work, no dental insurance, and little differential for working evenings or nights. It also means that many hospitals will require you to rotate shifts and to work more than half of the weekends.

You are not stupid. You know sick people need care around the clock, 7 days a week, 365 days a year, including weekends and holidays. However, you might not have considered what that would mean to *you* as a working nurse.

One hospital stated in its ad that "mandatory overtime" had been eliminated for nurses with 5 years of service. That means if you have been with the hospital less than 5 years, you will be required to work overtime.

In the late 1980s, hospitals were offering incentives such as job sharing, flexible schedules, sick child care, spa memberships, free maid service, and even sign-on bonuses of cold, hard cash.

By the end of 1993, many of these "perks" had disappeared. There were no sign-on bonuses, fewer flex time options, fewer educational opportunities. However, nursing continued to provide better-than-average benefits for both its full-time and *part-time* workers in important areas like health insurance, pension plans, sick days, and vacations than most other industries.

At the start of 1994, the average nurse, working full time in an acute care setting, was making about $40,000 a year. Starting salaries averaged between $32,000 and $34,000 a year. Inexperienced nurses made from $13 to $16 per hour; experienced nurses $17 to $24 per hour.

Compressed salary scales are less of a problem than they used to be. Five years ago, salary differences for inexperienced and experienced nurses varied as little as 10 to 15 percent. Today, there is a 30 percent difference. Other professions show a 50 percent difference, so we still have some catching up to do.

What will nursing be like by the time you graduate? There's only one way to find out. Come along for the ride.

4

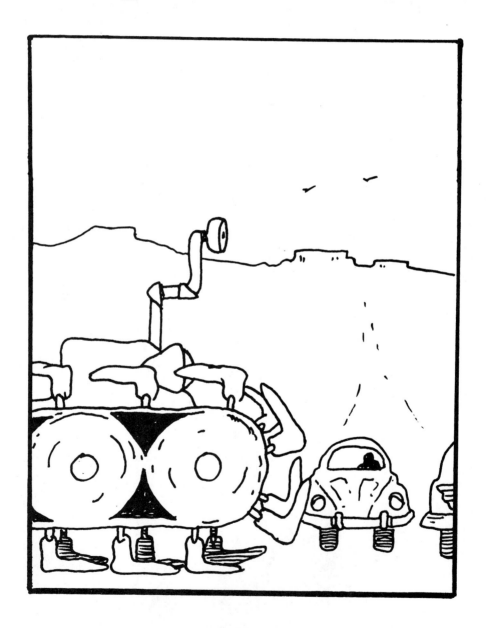

HOW LONG WILL THIS TRIP TAKE?

"Life is not one damn thing after another.
It's the same damn thing over and over."
—Edna St. Vincent Millay

When you first learned that there are three different routes (associate degree, diploma, baccalaureate) to becoming a registered nurse, you may have decided to take the fastest, cheapest, most convenient route. After all, who in his or her right mind would spend twice as much time and money to end up with the same credential? A nurse is a nurse.

That is like saying a car is a car. Although the statement is essentially true, it is not the whole truth. For example, both Volkswagen and Mercedes are fine automobiles. Either will provide you with years of dependable transportation. The Mercedes, however, comes equipped with many options not available on economy cars.

If you are enrolled in an associate degree or diploma program, you will emerge driving an economy car. Good job opportunities will be available for you, but some career opportunities will be inaccessible unless you "trade up."

Most hospital salary scales reinforce the nurse-is-a-nurse theory. Only 15 to 20 percent pay an R.N. with a bachelor's degree more than an R.N. without a bachelor's degree. However, those same hospitals often refuse to promote a staff nurse without a degree.

The debate over educational preparation for nurses has raged for decades and is hotly contested. It is the most divisive and potentially destructive issue facing nursing—which makes writing this chapter my most difficult challenge.

I have been a student in two of the three programs and a teacher in all of them. I would be the first to tell you that length of the program is no guarantee of quality. Admirable programs and abominable programs exist at every level. It is all in the engineering.

After you finish your education, you will be required to write a comprehensive set of exams to secure licensure as a registered nurse. To find how well your prospective nursing school is engineered, ask about its failure rates on State Board Examinations for the past 5 years. Until the last few years, a 5 percent failure rate meant "heads would roll"; the dean or director would be called on the carpet. By 1990 *average* failure rate approached 20 percent. Again, length of the program was not a factor. There were 2-year programs with a 0 percent failure rate and 4-year programs with a 37 percent failure rate. Make sure you go with a winner or your trip could take much longer than expected. In fact, you might never arrive!

As I said, writing this chapter has been my most difficult challenge. Actually, when I hit on the Mercedes/Volkswagen analogy, I thought it was a stroke of genius, a clever way to discuss the difference and keep with the book's theme.

After the first edition of this book hit the market, however, an instructor called to say she thought comparing her program to a VW was insulting. Ouch! I didn't choose the Mercedes-VW analogy to insult anyone. I chose it for clarity and because they are the only cars I have ever owned.

I was graduated from a diploma program in 1963 and bought a VW "Bug." That Bug served me well for thousands of miles and took me from the Midwest to the Northwest, where I got my bachelor's degree and my bachelor—Gary. We might still be driving Volkswagens today if things had not happened the way they did.

First, Gary's youngest brother was killed in an auto accident. Soon afterward a fellow graduate student was horribly injured in a crash. We became concerned about safety and believed we needed a more substantial car, but we were not sure what kind.

Buying the Mercedes began as a joke. We would go to the Mercedes showroom after dark and press our noses against the glass. One night the showroom was open. A supersalesman invited us in to view a film, which revealed safety features for the car that were incredible.

We were "sold," but we were poor graduate students. Not to worry! The dealer had a demonstrator at a great price, and he would give us a larger amount in trade-in allowance on the Bug than I had paid for it 4 years earlier. The dealer would even finance it. However, we were encouraged to see about bank financing because the dealer's was one-fourth of a percent higher.

The bankers laughed at us. We didn't have collateral, we had marginal incomes, and horror of horrors—what if I became pregnant?!? I assured them that was absolutely impossible because I was *already* pregnant. In fact, that was the reason we wanted a safer car.

Well, we bought that 1967 230S with dealer financing. Five months later we brought our newborn son home from the hospital in it. Both our sons grew up and learned to drive in that car. We drove it over 20 years and 280,000 miles until it finally succumbed to rust and teenage abuse. Today it lives on as an organ donor for a matching 230S we found a few years ago.

With cars, as with most things in life, it has been my experience that over the long run, the best often costs less. As you select a school of nursing, look to the long run. Think options and safety features.

LOOKING BEYOND THE HORIZON

It is not a question of becoming a nurse. All three paths lead *to* nursing. The question is, "What do you want to do *after* you become a nurse?" What sort of job would you like to have five years after graduation? Ten years after graduation?

At this stage of your journey, projecting yourself that far into the future may be nigh unto impossible. Just becoming a nurse seems light-years away. All you want to do is get that R.N. behind your name and get a job. Graduating from any nursing school will open the door to an excellent job. But some of you want a lot more than a job. Some of you already have very definite ideas of where you want to go once you reach nursing.

If you envision yourself as a public health nurse, clinical specialist, nurse practitioner, researcher, consultant, teacher, head nurse, or director of nursing services, you will need a baccalaureate degree. Yes, the *price* of a baccalaureate education is high, but the *cost* of not having one may be even higher. It all depends on where you want to go in nursing.

For most career-oriented nurses, a bachelor's degree is only the beginning. Many find that their chosen destination in nursing requires a trip to graduate school.

Our profession has lagged behind others in standardizing its educational requirements. Think about physical therapists, occupational therapists, dietitians, pharmacists, and social workers. All require the baccalaureate degree as minimal preparation, and many require a master's degree or above before full professional privileges are granted. For physicians, the baccalaureate degree is required before they are even eligible for entrance into their professional school. Nursing has some catching up to do.

What happens if you are an ADN or diploma graduate and somewhere down the road you decide you want more options? You take your "vehicle" back to the "factory" (college or university). Many colleges are purists. They will insist you cannot have a Mercedes chassis powered by a Volkswagen engine. They will offer to rebuild your vehicle completely if you can come up with enough money and approximately 3 more years of your life. Other colleges act more like body shops. They will be happy to customize your vehicle for less time and money.

Few students receive adequate counseling before choosing a school of nursing. They often learn about the advantages and disadvantages of their particular program in their *last semester.* Think carefully about the options you want and what you can "afford," not just in terms of dollars but in time and distance.

Actually, most of your instructors and many of the nurses you will come to admire are driving some of the most incredible contraptions you can imagine. Check their backgrounds and credentials. You will see that your basic preparation will not determine how far you can go in nursing, but it will affect the amount of time it takes to get there.

5

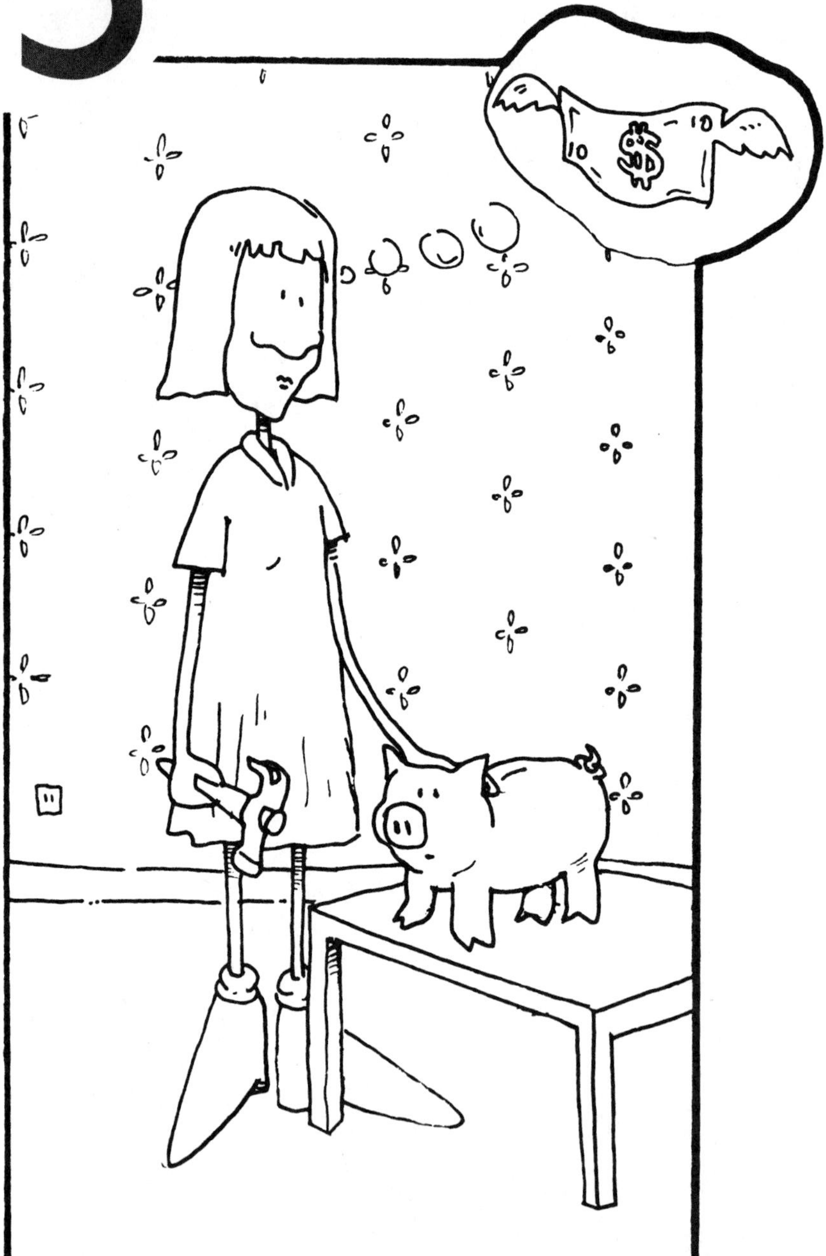

HOW MUCH WILL THIS TRIP COST?

"Look at me: I worked my way up from
nothing to a state of extreme poverty."
—Groucho Marx,
Monkey Business

Before starting any trip, it is wise to estimate the costs. Otherwise you may end up stranded and not only penniless, but deep in debt.

The costs of a nursing education vary widely. Checking the 1993 National League of Nursing numbers, you will find that a bachelor's degree in nursing can cost $1800 to $8000 per year, much more if you pay nonresident rates. Community colleges can cost $900 to $6800 per year, and diploma schools cost about $3400 a year.

These costs reflect tuition only. They do not include room and board and such miscellaneous costs as books, uniforms, special equipment, travel, and laboratory fees. Books, for example, cost an average of $400 per year. (Your first-year book bill may be significantly higher because many of the books required in the freshman year are used throughout the entire program.)

When estimating costs, don't forget to include such incidentals as transportation to and from the clinical area, babysitters, eating on the run, and a large bottle of aspirin.

One major cost often overlooked is that of deferred income—money you would have made if you had worked instead of going to school. If you allow $10,000 per year (a salary of $5 per hour), you can quickly see that the cost of *not working* will be $20,000 or $30,000 or $40,000, depending on whether you are enrolled in an associate degree, diploma, or baccalaureate program.

How much will *your* trip to nursing cost? Sit down with your classmates and discuss all the potential costs, including deferred income. Work through the following exercise. The total figure will be quite a jolt.

Cost estimates of spending _____ years at _____
school of nursing

Tuition   _____

Room and board   _____

Books   _____

Uniform/special equipment   _____

Laboratory fees   _____

Transportation   _____

Deferred income   _____

Other:

_____   _____

_____   _____

_____   _____

TOTAL   _____

Of course, there are ways to defray costs. You may be eligible for a scholarship, grant, or loan. Usually scholarships are given for academic achievement, whereas grants are based strictly on financial need. Student loans tend to carry very low interest charges, and repayment is not required until after graduation. Unlike loans, scholarships and grants do not have to be repaid.

MEGABUCKS IN MOTION

To find money to help finance your education, ask local hospitals, auxiliaries, nursing associations, service clubs, and fraternal orders about their scholarship programs. Check the public library. Even if you are 40 years old, call your local high school counselor for advice. Don't forget the armed forces. They have some excellent scholarship and financial aid benefits. Valuable information may also be obtained by contacting the National League for Nursing, the American Nurses' Association (ANA), your state chapter of the ANA, the National Student Nurses' Association, and the Canadian Nurses' Association. (Addresses are in Appendixes F and G.)

Monies are available from both the public and the private sectors. Since eligibility requirements and dollar amounts change annually, your best source of current information will be the financial aid office at your nursing school. You may also be eligible for a work-study program. Remember, just because you didn't start with a scholarship, grant, or loan doesn't mean you can't get one. Some monies become available only after you complete lower-division courses. Appendix D contains addresses you need to find out more about undergraduate financial aid and student loan programs.

Nursing students have taken out second mortgages, borrowed against insurance policies, and sold their boats, cars, and motorcycles to finance their education. A middle-aged student got a loan from her mother because "Mom always wanted me to become a nurse and she thought it was better late than never!" Another student said she was in school on "found" money. Once she decided to go to school, she found there were a lot of things she could do without.

Most of you are comparison shoppers. You try to get top value for each dollar spent. You watch for sales, clip coupons, and drive miles out of the way to save a few bucks.

When it comes to educational dollars, however, some students behave in a most irrational manner. They would never dream of going to the store and asking the clerk, "What's the least I can get for 20 bucks?" Yet they plunk their tuition money down and then ask the instructor, "What's the least I can get for this and still graduate?" They concentrate on the *minimum* requirements instead of reaching for the *maximum.*

Regardless of what financial aid you manage to muster, this educational experience is still going to cost you thousands and thousands of dollars. So approach education in a businesslike manner. You have "contracted" with the school for certain services. Make sure it delivers. You have "hired" these instructors. Be sure to get what you have paid for by learning and experiencing everything you can.

Be a smart consumer. Get your money's worth.

The cost of a nursing education cannot be measured in dollars alone. There is another price that will be paid in blood, sweat, and tears.

NOW THEY KNOW

I asked students attending a National Student Nurses' Association convention to share one thing they wish they had known before deciding to major in nursing. Here are some of their answers:

"ONE THING I WISH I HAD KNOWN *BEFORE* I CHOSE TO MAJOR IN NURSING IS

> . . . how difficult it was going to be!"
> . . . how much reading there is."
> . . . how much paperwork there is to do!"
> . . . that so much outside work was required."
> . . . that even though I was an honor student in high school, college is totally different."
> . . . how much actual work it requires! (Or maybe I'm glad I didn't know. I might not have finished.)"
> . . . that I would need to keep white underwear in stock for the rest of my life."

... how to prepare for the shock and trauma of the nursing class/clinical schedule."

... that fraternities may have 'Hell Week' but nursing has 'Hell Years.' "

... the astonishing amount of knowledge you must gain in 4 years."

... what nursing really is."

... what nurses really do."

... more about the three different ways to become an R.N."

... all about the entry into practice issue! I certainly would have appreciated the honesty."

... the expense!"

... that you are no longer an individual until you graduate—you belong to the nursing program, physically and spiritually. On graduation you develop wings and fly."

... the number of clinical options available."

... how much time I would be investing (I'm married) and how much discipline I would need (and how much weight I was going to gain!)."

6

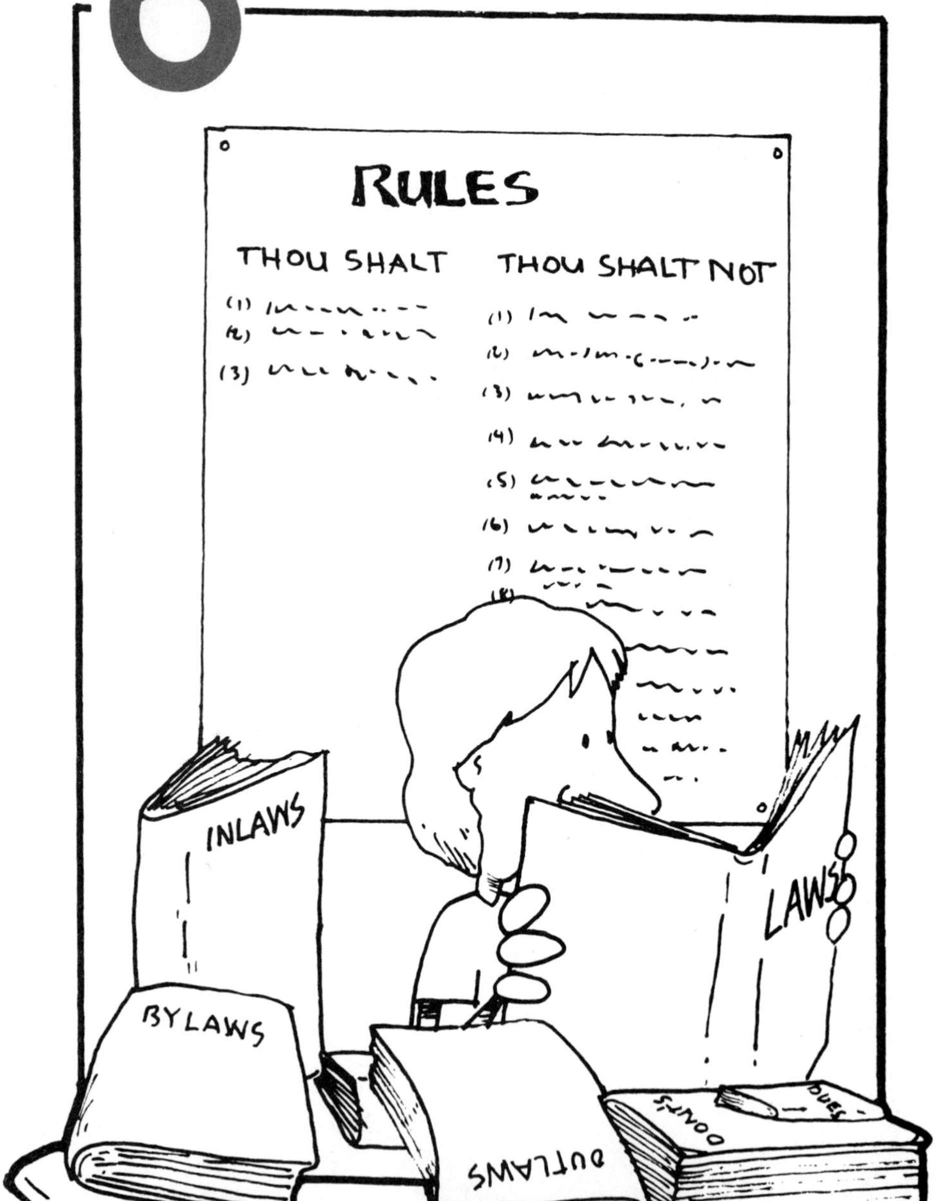

RULES
THOU SHALT
THOU SHALT NOT
INLAWS
LAWS
BYLAWS
OUTLAWS
DON'TS
DUES

RULES OF THE ROAD

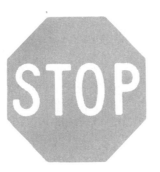

"Each is given a bag of tools,
A shapeless mass,
A book of rules;
And each must make,
Ere life is flown,
A stumbling-block
Or a stepping-stone."
—R. L. Sharpe
Stumbling-Block or Stepping-Stone

All schools of nursing are similar, but no two are identical. Each has designed its own highly customized track on which you will learn how to be a nurse.

Upon your admission, the school effectively issues you a learner's permit. If you fail to follow the rules of *its* road, your permit may be canceled. Therefore knowing the rules and regulations is imperative.

So . . . READ THE RULES. Take two aspirin and read them again. Ignorance can cost you big bucks and add months to your program. Don't be caught saying, "I didn't know . . . I had to have organic chemistry first . . . my incomplete would automatically convert to an F . . . Abnormal Psychology was only offered winter quarter . . . three clinical absences meant I had to repeat the course . . . advanced registration began last week . . . fees were due Monday."

Check the college catalog, the student handbook, special orientation packets, and all first-day-of-class handouts. Don't just read them, study them. Underline vital information and make notes in the margins. Highlight those things that apply to you immediately or in the near future. If you have questions, get clarification. Don't rely on the grapevine for the latest word on course requirements. Go directly to the source. Talk with the instructor involved.

These policies were not written by God, but they might as well have been. They do not reflect spur-of-the-moment decisions. They are decisions that have evolved over many years. Countless deans, directors, faculty members, students, advisory boards, and ad hoc committees have devised and revised the rules and regulations governing your school of nursing.

If the rules and regulations begin to get you down, remember that what appears to be a roadblock may actually be a guardrail placed there to keep you from plunging off a cliff.

RULES AND REASONS

Schools of nursing represent a huge investment in manpower and machinery. Their programs are among the most expensive to run. They are insured to the hilt and are accountable to more governmental and professional agencies than you can imagine. They will supply you with teachers, classrooms, laboratories, disposable equipment, and not-so-disposable patients. The schools shoulder an enormous responsibility. In return you must grant them a few eccentricities.

For example, most schools have written codes for dress and behavior. This irks the daylights out of some students. They consider it an infringement on their personal rights.

It is nothing personal. It is strictly professional. This may be the first time your personal freedoms collide with professional responsibilities, but it won't be the last.

Before bursting into a chorus of "I've Gotta Be Me," consider the advantages of being "me" on your own time. You can avoid all sorts of headaches and hassles if you simply agree to bathe regularly, use deodorant, buy a bra, trim your beard, wear shoes, spit out your chewing gum, or give up earrings that dangle in your soup.

On the school's time, be a polished professional. On your own time, cut loose, relax, and enjoy. At first you may feel absolutely schizophrenic. Gradually, the "real" you and the "professional" you will meld and mature into a "new" you.

If you want to stay in school, CONFORM. Sure, you can fight the system. But face it, you don't have the time, energy, or cunning it takes to win. You'll just end up spinning your wheels while other students drive off with diplomas.

Instead of fighting the system, use it. When conflicts arise, take your concerns, suggestions, and grievances to the student-faculty committee responsible for such matters. Then hurry back to the business of learning. After all, your job is not to revamp this school of nursing. Your job is to graduate.

There is no such thing as a perfect school of nursing, an optimum curriculum, or an ideal textbook. But we are working on it. That is why you will find curricula constantly under construction, courses being remodeled, textbooks being switched mid-year, and learning experiences that seem to appear and disappear without warning. Be sure to see your advisor regularly to be aware of any upcoming changes as well as to keep tabs on your progress.

One student inquired about a computer course labeled 108X. Although the description sounded like just what she needed, she noticed no other course in that column had an "X rating." She was told it denoted an experimental course that was "not quite approved." She wisely chose another course that was fully approved.

When you are handed an armload of paper listing miles of rules and regulations, it is hard to believe all this has been compiled to make student life *less* complicated. On careful examination, however, you'll find that these papers do more than outline your obligations—they safeguard your opportunities. Following the instructions makes your graduation not only a possibility but a distinct probability.

Yes, there are exceptions to every rule. But are you really that exceptional?

> "This is the grave of Mike O'Day
> Who died maintaining his right of way.
> His right was clear, his will was strong,
> But he's just as dead as if he'd been wrong."
> —*Epitaph*

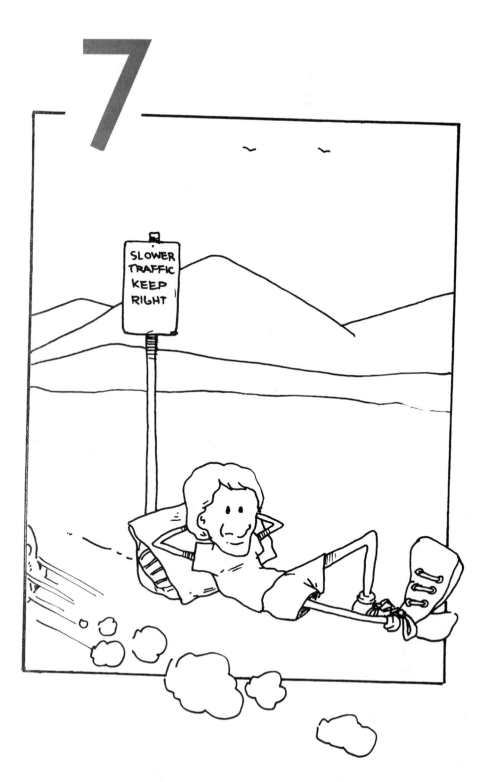

SLOWER TRAFFIC KEEP RIGHT

SLOWER TRAFFIC KEEP RIGHT

"Too swift arrives as tardy as too slow."
—Shakespeare,
Romeo and Juliet

If you are just starting out on your first lap around the track, listen to some student-to-student tips for success. Students attending a National Student Nurses' Association convention were asked to share one "survival" tip they would like to pass on to beginning students.

Their suggestions can be divided into four categories: (1) take care of yourself; (2) take care of each other; (3) take one day at a time; and (4) take care of business.

TAKE CARE OF YOURSELF

"Set time aside each day for yourself or your family."

"Don't spend all of your time studying."

"Make sure to take care of yourself. Don't put nursing school ahead of your own health."

"Make sure you look your best every day. The better you look, the better others will treat you."

"Take a fun elective."

"Study hard, but play hard too. Make time for friends. Take walks, work out, dance, swim, play tennis—it will keep you sane."

SLOWER
TRAFFIC
KEEP
RIGHT

TAKE CARE OF EACH OTHER

"Build a support system with your fellow students."

"Work together as a class. Don't let the competitive spirit get in the way."

"Get involved early with NSNA. Networking is important."

"Join a study group. I couldn't have made it without mine."

"Study with friends. Try studying for 50 minutes and playing or talking for 10 minutes. Repeat. It's not much of a social life, but it's better than nothing."

"Get involved with other students. They can help you, and you can help them."

TAKE ONE DAY AT A TIME

"Take it one day, one test, one patient at a time, and don't get discouraged."

"Don't take introductory classes too seriously. They are meant to weed out students. Hang in there until clinical. You'll love it!"

"Live one day at a time. Once something is done, don't worry about it. Just keep doing your best at each task."

"Make the best of any situation by adjusting *your* attitude."

"Please yourself—be happy meeting your own personal/ professional/academic goals."

"Looking at the overall picture can be pretty scary. Just concentrate on one assignment at a time."

TAKE CARE OF BUSINESS

"MAKE NURSING SCHOOL YOUR FIRST PRIORITY."

"Take classes seriously. Start out studying hard."

"Maintain good study habits."

"Keep up with the reading from Day One."

"Do the reading as you go along. Don't wait!"

"Take the extra time needed to do extra readings."

"KEEP UP WITH WORK RATHER THAN TRYING TO CATCH UP."

"Start a good home library to use for care plans."

"Keep your notes current."

"Review notes daily."

"Organize your time. Conserve your energy."

"Use Sunday night to plan your entire week."

"Create your own flash cards."

"Be prepared for three times more work than you ever imagined."

"Take a course in stress management."

"Build up your GPA before you start taking all nursing courses."

"Learn to be happy with Cs and thrilled with Bs (especially if you were a straight-A student in high school)."

"Get a tutor if necessary."

"Do not take too many sciences in one semester."

"Make sure you're financially stable enough to work minimal hours while in school."

"Realize that it is impossible to work full time and be a good student. If you want to survive nursing, don't try to work full time."

"Get to know your instructors."

"Do what the teacher tells you to do. Don't argue; just do it! It will decrease your stress and your teacher's stress too."

"Buy a book on nursing math and bone up ahead of time."

"Don't just memorize material. Learn how to apply it."

"KEEP YOUR SENSE OF HUMOR!"

"Learn how to live without sleep."

"Don't forget to breathe."

Ready? Set? Go! Take the on ramp and don't look back. Just go slowly and stay in the right lane.

8

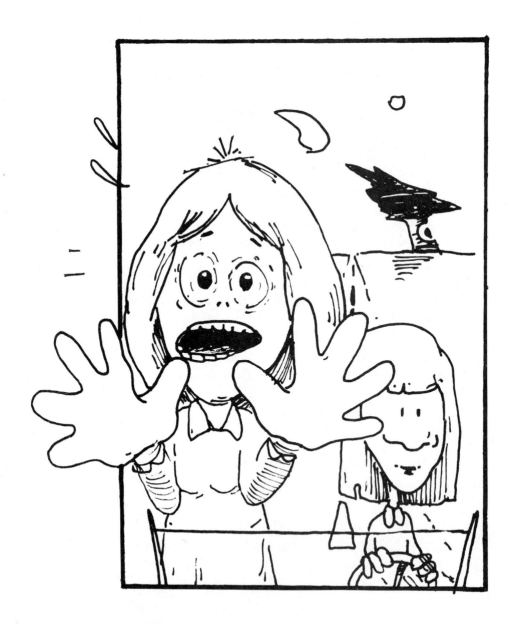

DRIVING INSTRUCTORS

SCHOOL

"You know how I'm smart? I got people around me who know more than I do."
—Louis B. Mayer

Meet your driving instructors. These are the experts you've hired to take you over the course. Get to know them. Remember that they are people first, nurses second, and teachers third.

Get to know them as people. They are human. They are not infallible, omniscient, or omnipotent. They have their likes and dislikes, their dreams and fears, their good days and bad days, their strengths and weaknesses. They have diverse cultural, familial, religious, and geographic backgrounds. Each has a different philosophy of life.

Get to know them as nurses. Find out what attracted them to nursing in the first place, where they were educated, what their clinical specialties are, where they have worked, which professional organizations they belong to, what articles or books they have written, and what their goals are. Each has a different philosophy of nursing.

Get to know them as teachers. Find out how long they have been teaching, where else they have taught, what their favorite subject matter is, and in which clinical areas they enjoy guiding students. Some instructors see themselves as scholars and researchers. Others see themselves as catalysts, facilitators, role models, or even recruiters for the nursing profession. Each has a different philosophy of teaching.

Your goal is not to "psych out" the instructors so you can get by with learning as little as possible. Your goal is to "psych out" the instructors so you can learn as *much* as possible.

CHOICE INSTRUCTORS

By identifying instructors compatible with your needs, goals, philosophy, and style, you can make learning much easier. For example, if you prefer freedom to examine, experience, and discover information for yourself, you will suffocate under an instructor who delivers formal lectures and insists that everyone stay together in lock-step fashion. On the other hand, if you are a student who prefers a lot of structure and no surprises, you might excel under such an instructor.

Avoid instructors with whom you are dreadfully mismatched in terms of style, philosophy, or temperament. If you find yourself in such a situation, decide whether you can successfully adapt or should seek an immediate transfer. Avoid any instructor who boasts of being a harsh grader. Always remember that your Number One Goal is to graduate.

Keep your eyes open for instructors who are masters of their craft, intellectually stimulating, and accessible in times of trouble. Instructors are prone to clone, so stick close to those you would like to resemble when you grow up (professionally speaking).

"A teacher affects eternity; he can never tell where his influence stops."
—Henry Adams,
The Education of Henry Adams

Most instructors hold advanced degrees and, in the course of obtaining those degrees, have become highly specialized. That is why teaching teams are so common in schools of nursing. A team of instructors picks you up at point X and delivers you to point Y, where another team of specialists takes over. It's rather like a cross between a road rally and a relay race.

ONE FOR THE ROAD

Whenever you encounter a new set of instructors, always assume the best. "These instructors are here to help me. They sincerely want me to succeed. They will do everything they can in my behalf." Even in the face of evidence to the contrary, assume the best.

Positive attitudes are contagious. Instructors enjoy working with students who are optimistic, courteous, cooperative, self-disciplined, responsible, respectful, and proud of the work they are doing. The more of these attributes you have, the more successful you will be.

Negative attitudes are equally contagious. If you are pessimistic, uncooperative, hesitant, or uninterested, your nonverbal behavior will give away your inner thoughts. The instructors will have an uneasy feeling about you. They will begin to question your ability, and your chances of failure will be greater.

Your relationship with your nursing instructors will mirror your relationships with authority figures in general. Think about how you relate to parents, clergy, employers, police officers, and other authorities. Do you see them as friends or foes? Are you usually agreeable or argumentative? Suspicious or trusting?

There are only two totally unreasonable nursing instructors in the entire country. Invariably, one will be employed by your school of nursing. If you think you are dealing with more than one totally unreasonable instructor, *you* have a problem. You are either in the wrong school, the wrong profession, or both.

TEACHER/LEARNER/STUDENT/NURSE

You may be surprised to learn that many of your nursing instructors are students themselves. Many are working on advanced degrees. They have to write term papers and take final exams. They have to worry about their own GPAs as well as yours.

Just as the nursing profession is moving toward standardizing its educational requirements to be on a par with other professions, nursing education is moving toward requiring the same credentials held by college professors in other departments.

Only a few years ago in many schools of nursing, a bachelor's degree was considered adequate preparation for many teaching positions. Today, teaching opportunities for nurses with bachelor's degrees are few and fleeting. Occasionally these nurses are hired to help teach in the clinical setting on a temporary basis. For most faculty members a master's degree is required, and doctoral preparation is preferred. At many colleges and universities, master's-prepared nurses are being phased out unless they are actively working toward a doctorate.

Having to be teacher and graduate student simultaneously is only one pressure felt by nursing faculty. In addition to their teaching duties, nursing faculty are also expected to engage in research, to publish widely, to be politically active, to perform community service, and to maintain competence in their clinical area. Try adding marriage and/or children to all of this and you have a better understanding of why faculty members are not always as accessible or patient as you would like them to be.

ROLES ROYCE

On the rocky road through nursing, your instructors will play many roles. As TOUR GUIDES they will plan the itinerary, provide maps, and staff the information booth. They will lead you through unfamiliar territory, introducing you to local customs, acting as interpreters, and making sure you don't offend the natives. Since they know what's coming around each bend, they will make sure you don't miss anything. By sharing stories and anecdotes, they weave together the past, present, and future of nursing.

As CONSTRUCTION WORKERS they pave the way so you can pass quickly and safely. They flag you around potholes and other possible pitfalls. They fill in gaps, build bridges, and lay good foundations. They know that before new structures can be built, old ones sometimes must be de-

molished. They help you bulldoze old attitudes, habits, preju-
dices, and other misinformation.

As HIGHWAY PATROL OFFICERS they police the road
for your patient's protection. They not only handle emergencies and accidents, they also help prevent them by enforcing
rules and regulations. They make sure everyone is going in
the right direction at the right speed. If you break the rules,
they may let you off with a warning or they may issue a formal citation that lands you in front of the judge.

As TRAFFIC COURT JUDGES they listen to individual
cases and hear appeals. They may place you on probation,
fine you, or suspend your license to learn. Not all of an instructor's tasks are pleasant, but all are necessary.

9

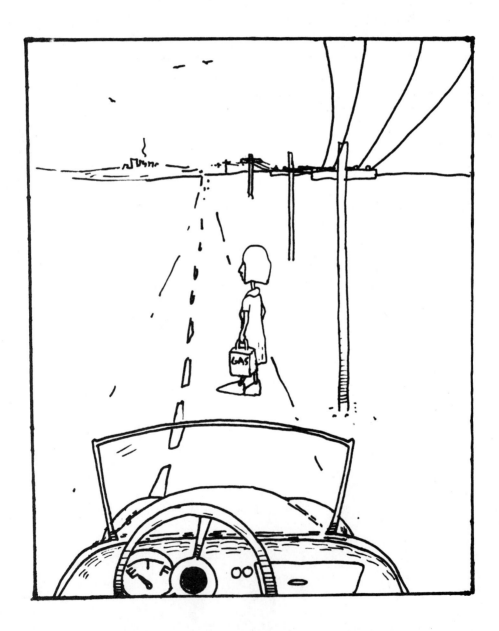

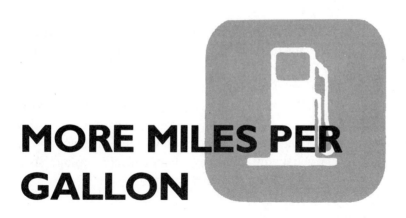

MORE MILES PER GALLON

"Genius is one percent inspiration and
ninety-nine percent perspiration."
—Thomas Edison

Think of the hours in your week as gallons of gas in your tank. Every student has precisely the same amount, yet some get much farther on their weekly tank of gas than others.

If you want to get more miles per gallon, there are two things you must do. You must learn to be more EFFICIENT and more EFFECTIVE. Being more efficient means learning to do things right. Being more effective means learning to do the right things.

When it comes to efficiency, you can get more mileage by improving your reading and writing skills than any other way. Do whatever is necessary to increase your proficiency (see "Reading and Remembering" in Chapter 12). These skills will not only bring success for you as a student, they will also give you the leading edge as a professional in years to come.

Front-running students know how to conserve fuel. They know that the difference between studying for short periods and studying for long periods is like the difference between city and highway driving. They know they will accomplish more, faster, and with less wear and tear on their machinery if they take studying up to cruising speed and hold it there for an hour, or two, or three.

43

But no matter how efficient you become, you still will not get where you want to go if you drive off in the wrong direction. That is where effectiveness comes into play. You not only need to read well, you need to read right—the right books, the right chapters, the right journals. You may be a faster writer and technically flawless yet write wrong—the wrong topics, the wrong themes, the wrong conclusions.

How do you know what's right and what's wrong? Ask your instructor. Listen carefully.

IMPROVING YOUR FUEL EFFICIENCY

Another way students manage to get more miles to the gallon is by driving economical models. They operate under a principle described by an ancient Italian economist named Pareto. His 80/20 principle, loosely translated, says that 80 percent of the value or satisfaction will come from 20 percent of the tasks or activities.

So if you have 10 things to do today, two of them will account for 80 percent of the day's success. Leading students are able to look at their "*to do*" list and zero in on the two or three activities that have the highest payoff potential. They tackle those first. If there is time left, they take care of some of the remaining items.

Floundering students make no distinction regarding the payoff value of items on their to do lists. They begin anywhere, usually with the easiest items. By the end of the day they have accomplished eight of the 10 items on their list. Unfortunately, they did the eight that gave them only a 20 percent return on their time.

Using this proportional approach when setting priorities has some very practical applications. For example, if your instructor is a specialist in the subject matter, 80 percent of the test will come from lecture and only 20 percent will come from the readings. However, if the instructor is a specialist in cardiac care but has to pinch-hit in a psychiatric nursing course, 80 percent of the test will come from the readings and only 20 percent will come from lecture.

Once you become aware of the 80/20 principle, you will begin to see all sorts of other applications. You will notice that

80 percent of your homework comes from 20 percent of your teachers; that 80 percent of all prescriptions involve only 20 percent of the drugs; and that 80 percent of what you need to know is contained in 20 percent of your textbook. Ah . . . if only you knew which 20 percent!

Superstudents have developed the ability to pick out the 20 percent of the reading that gives them 80 percent of what they need to know. The don't try to master everything in the textbook. They concentrate on that small percentage that allows them to sail through exams and to perform competently in the clinical area. If you need help developing this ability, see Chapter 12, "Drive-Up Teller."

Here are some other tips to help you get more miles per gallon.

TIME MANAGEMENT FROM A TO Z FOR NURSING STUDENTS

ATTENDANCE. Every hour you spend in class will save you 3 hours of study time. If you are going to cut corners somewhere, go to class and skimp on study time. Attend every class.

BUDGETING. Most students claim they just don't have enough time. Yet every student has all the time there is: 168 hours per week, no more and no less. Therefore managing your time becomes even more important than managing your money because once time is spent, you can't earn more.

To make sure you use each day to the maximum, buy a pocket-sized daily planner and keep it with you. Buy a jumbo calendar to keep track of major events. Scope the whole term, marking out such milestones as exams, term papers, and research projects. Block out all clinical times. Don't forget to allow time for preclinical work such as reading charts, making care plans, and interviewing patients.

Approach being a student as you would a job. Plan to be at it 40 hours a week. Small-business owners will tell you they average closer to 60 hours a week, and you qualify as a *small* business.

Don't make the mistake of thinking that because you have only one class on Tuesday and no class on Thursday, those are your "days off." Actually, those are the days when you can really get down to business; although it is important to use every fragment of time, it is even more important to schedule large blocks of uninterrupted study time lasting 2 or 3 hours.

CONCENTRATION. One key to success is undivided attention. Eliminate all distractions. Clear your work area and your mind of all clutter. Keep on the desk only what you need for a particular assignment. If your mind wanders, order it back to the task at hand. Superstudents not only do first things first, they do only one thing at a time.

DIRTY JOBS. Look at your "to-do-today" list and circle the task you dread doing most. Tackle that one first. When it is finished, you will feel exhilarated.

If you postpone doing a boring, tough, or unpleasant task, it will nag you all day. Your ability to concentrate will be nil. As the day wears on, you will begin to think about putting it off until tomorrow. That way the task will ruin 2 days instead of 1. So take the plunge and do the dirty job first.

EQUIPMENT. Have a ready supply of pens, pencils, paper, notecards, computer disks, and printer ribbons on hand. There is nothing more inconvenient than having to make a mad dash to an all-night convenience store.

Invest in the latest edition of each required textbook. Should you buy a used book? Buying a pre-owned book is like buying a used car. If the previous owner was a straight-A student, the yellow highlights and scribbles in the margins may be a godsend. Unfortunately, most straight-A students keep their books. The market is flooded with C-minus students' books. If your eye is easily distracted, buy a new one.

To avoid frequent trips to the library for minor tidbits of information, build your own mini-reference library.

Besides a standard dictionary and thesaurus, include a medical/nursing dictionary, drug handbook, *Merck Medical Manual*, and _____. (Ask your instructors for suggestions to fill in the blank.)

FILING SYSTEM. With the "it-must-be-here-somewhere" filing system, you will not only lose time, you will lose your temper. Browse at the local bookstore for a filing system that meets your needs. If you can't afford what's in the store, go behind the store and get a sturdy cardboard box from the trash. Keep everything together. Put all papers pertaining to a certain class in one folder, and keep all folders for the current term in one box.

Once the term is over, take all those folders and move them to an under-the-bed storage box. That way the stuff will be out of sight but easily accessible. Then when your classroom studies are focused on the renal system but you find yourself caring for a pregnant schizophrenic with a broken leg, you can quickly find your notes from last term or even last year.

GOALS. Goals may be as simple as reading two chapters before bedtime or as complex as becoming a nurse-midwife in Borneo. Some take 10 minutes to accomplish; others take 10 years.

Being goal oriented helps you focus your time and energy for maximum effect. It enables you to weed out irrelevant people and activities. Dozens of daily decisions become automatic.

If you find yourself wishing you could get a better grade in anatomy and physiology, or get into the clinical rotation at Children's Hospital next spring, or get more help with the housework, stop wishing and convert those wishes into goals. Sit down and work through the following:

1. List the steps you need to take to achieve the goal.
2. Decide which steps you are *able* to take to achieve the goal.
3. Decide which steps you are *willing* to take to achieve the goal.

4. Identify people who can help you achieve the goal.
5. Consider how you might let yourself or others sabotage your good intentions.

If you take the time to write down a goal and your plan for achieving it, you won't need a fairy godmother to make your dreams come true.

HANGING IN THERE. When the going gets tough, hang in there. As the difficulty of any task increases, so does the attractiveness of *any* distraction. As you squirm in your chair, doing your laundry suddenly seems vital. Ignore the laundry. Knuckle down and work through the problem at hand. If you abandon a task when you feel you are losing, you'll find it much harder to return to it. Active avoidance coupled with passive procrastination will cost you lots of time. Instead, stop work at a point where you feel you are winning. Then you will be willing, even eager, to return to the task later.

INVESTMENTS. Think of class attendance, library time, and study sessions as "deposits." Even brief moments, like small change, can add up to something big. One student tucked chemical formulas into her ski boot and memorized them on the chairlift.

Learn to prioritize. Invest time in high-payoff activities. Required classes take priority over electives. Nursing classes take priority over any other class. Studying for an exam that makes up 50 percent of your grade takes precedence over studying for an exam that only makes up 10 percent of a grade. And so on.

JOTTING IT DOWN. Make lists and use them. It's the best way to keep organized and avoid wasted motion. Lists help you consolidate errands so that you make two trips instead of twenty. Lists help you arrive prepared and ready for action.

Efficiency experts suggest you make a list each evening for the following day. List the six most critical things that have to be done. Rank them in order of importance. The next day, begin with Number One and work it through before going on to anything else. Continue down the list. Your productivity will skyrocket.

KNOCKING OFF. When you reach the point of diminishing returns, discontinue an activity. Settle for an A—don't knock your brains out striving for an A-plus. No one wastes more time than a perfectionist.

Remember Parkinson's Law: "Work expands to fill the amount of time available to do it." Set reasonable deadlines and stick to them. Then move on to the next task.

LIBRARIAN. No one on campus can help you save as much time as the librarian. Just ask.

MAJORING IN MINOR ACTIVITIES. Busywork gives many students a false sense of accomplishment. Each night they fall into bed exhausted, insisting they are working as hard as they can. They're right. They're just not working as *smart* as they can.

Learn to recognize busywork for what it is. Don't take pride in your efforts. Take pride only in results.

"NO." The greatest time-saving device ever invented.

OTHER PEOPLE'S TIME. Time-wise students know how to divide chores and delegate everything they possibly can. They are also aware of some important considerations when relying on other people's time.

For example, if you are hiring someone to type your term paper, get the material to the typist well in advance of the due date. One campus typist, tired of last-minute hysterics, posted this notice on her wall: "A LACK OF PLANNING ON YOUR PART DOES NOT CONSTI-

TUTE AN EMERGENCY ON MINE." If you are relying on other people's time, plan *far* ahead.

PRIME TIME. Every person has 2 or 3 hours a day when he or she is in top form. Most of us have our prime time in the morning.

Find your prime time and protect it. Invest it in high-priority items that demand concentration, creativity, and judgment. Use your less-than-prime time for legwork.

QUESTIONS. Several times each day, ask yourself questions such as the following:

- Is this the best use of my time right now?
- Is this activity helping me achieve one of my goals?
- Is this worth the amount of time it will take?
- Is this still worth doing?
- If I didn't do this, what would happen?

REGRETS. Don't squander time mourning what might have been. Don't waste time wallowing in guilt or self-pity. When you begin to say, "If only _____," quickly change the statement to "Next time _____." Then get on with the business at hand.

SAVING TIME. Impossible! It is also impossible to *find* time or *make* time. You can only put the time you have to better use.

TOMORROW. It never comes. Do it TODAY.

URGENCY! Urgent things are not always important. Important things are not always urgent. Tending to the important and ignoring the pseudoimportant things that clamor for attention are what separate good students from great students.

VACILLATING. Indecision robs students of enough time to be classified as grand larceny. Be decisive. Establish your own operating policies. If you give yourself a deadline, stick to it. If you decide your regular study period will be from 2 to 4 P.M. Monday through Friday, don't violate that policy. Studying anything is better than studying nothing.

WASTEBASKET. Use it!

XEROXING. For dimes and quarters you can cut your library time to the bone. Use your less-than-prime time to round up all appropriate books and journals. Scan 2 minutes for articles, 3 minutes for books. Photocopy anything that appears pertinent. Use your prime time to study, memorize, integrate, synthesize, and use the information.

Keep copies of all your written papers and major assignments. It's a dirt-cheap insurance policy against loss.

YAKETY YAK. Don't let the telephone or a drop-in visitor ruin your study time. Tell callers, "I can't talk right now. I'll call you back at 9 o'clock." If you can't do that, unplug the phone or go where there are no phones.

Close your door. If someone pops in and asks, "Have you got a minute," say "No, but I'll have a minute at 9 o'clock." Offer to meet in his or her room or in the coffee shop. That way you can control the length of the visit.

ZZZZS. Schedule rest-and-relaxation periods. Get the sleep you need so you will be alert enough to put all these time-management suggestions to good use.

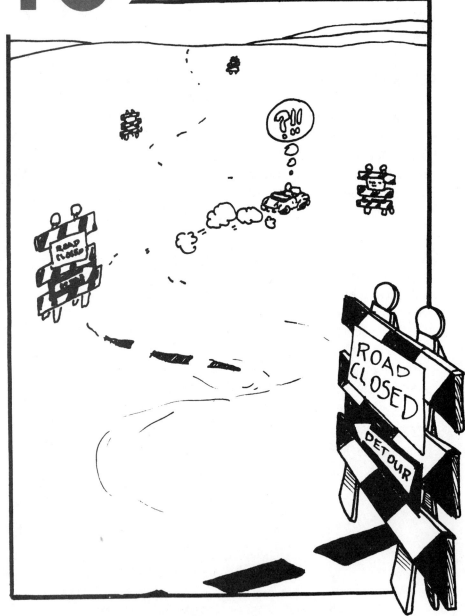

DETOURS

"Lost time is never found again."
—Benjamin Franklin,
Poor Richard's Almanac

Clutching your "THINGS TO DO" list, you start off with the best intentions. Today you are really going to cover ground. There is a term paper to tackle, a chemistry quiz coming up, a patient to interview, some assigned journal articles to read, and a dental appointment at 3 o'clock. But first you'd better throw in a load of laundry (DETOUR). Then the phone rings (DETOUR).

Finally you are off and running. Rounding the first bend, you bump into an old friend who invites you for coffee (DETOUR). Now 2 hours behind schedule, you arrive at the library. Looking for the required journal articles, you happen upon a fascinating issue about career planning (DETOUR). That leaves time to read only three of the required articles before class.

After class you walk over to the hospital and find that your patient is unavailable. (He is always in physical therapy at this time of day.) Oh well, you can kill some time in the cafeteria (DETOUR).

The patient interview takes longer than you expected, making you 15 minutes late for class. Embarrassed to walk in late, you decide to cut class (DETOUR). You go directly to chem lab and begin preparing for today's assignment.

Leaving lab a few minutes early, you dash to the dentist's office. You are on time, but he isn't. You are kept waiting for an hour. Unfortunately, you left your chemistry notes at the lab, so you decide to write a long-overdue letter to your mom (DETOUR).

With half your face numb, you leave the dentist's office. You drive toward campus intending to start work on that term paper. Caught in rush-hour traffic, you suddenly feel drained. It has been a long day. You deserve an evening off. You turn around and head for home thinking, "There's always tomorrow" (DETOUR).

KNOW THE WARNING SIGNS

The word *detour* comes from the French meaning "to divert." Diversions come in all shapes, sizes, and disguises. Keeping on course requires constant attention. To avoid unnecessary detours, ask yourself several times a day: "Is what I am doing or about to do helping me reach one of my goals?" If the answer is no, you are on a detour.

Most students who fail to graduate aren't losers, they just get lost. They start out on the right road but forget where they are going. They lose sight of their goal. They are lured off the track by seemingly harmless diversions.

Always keep your eye on the finish line. Never forget that your NUMBER ONE GOAL IS TO GRADUATE.

Goals determine priorities. Priorities determine how you allocate such limited resources as time, money, and energy. Graduation is your long-term goal. All of your short-term goals should contribute directly or indirectly to that end.

The only way to graduate is to stay in school. The only way to stay in school is to successfully complete one test, one paper, one patient, one clinical skill, one term at a time. These are the minor goals that add up to your major goal.

WISHBONES VERSUS BACKBONES

Students spend a lot of time wishing:

"I wish my term paper were done."
"I wish I could lose 10 pounds."

"I wish I didn't procrastinate so much."
"I wish I could get a better grade in chemistry."
"I wish my family helped more with household chores."
"I wish I could get into a different clinical group."

Converting a wish into a goal requires a workable plan. To formulate such a plan, ask yourself the five following questions:

1. What do I need to do to get what I want?
2. What am I *willing* to do to get what I want?
3. How will getting what I want affect my life?
4. Who can I count on to help me get what I want?
5. How might I sabotage myself so I don't get what I want?

Let's take "I wish I could get a better grade in chemistry" and work it through from a wish to a goal.

1. **What do I need to do to get a better grade in chemistry?**

I might need to do such things as:

- Spend extra time studying chemistry assignments.
- Memorize formulas.
- Ask questions in class.
- Complete all assignments.
- Join a study group.
- Hire a tutor.
- Buy a study guide or supplementary textbook.
- Change lab partners.
- Ask the instructor for help.
- Do projects for extra credit.

2. **What am I willing to do to get a better grade in chemistry?**

Reading over the list I made in response to the first question, I circle those things I am willing and able to do to improve my grade. I will be scrupulously honest. There is no sense trying to kid myself.

Knowing what has to be done and doing it are two different things. If I refuse to take the steps I have outlined, getting a better grade in chemistry remains a wish and never becomes a goal.

3. How will getting a better grade in chemistry affect my life?

If I know what I have to do to get a better grade but am unwilling to take the necessary action, this question might give me the extra incentive I need. The results may be worth the effort if by improving my grade I can keep from flunking out, or raise my GPA, or increase my self-esteem and confidence.

Since I cannot "find" time or "make" time, I am going to have to "take" time away from other activities. Shifting time to chemistry may mean getting up an hour earlier or going to bed an hour later. It may mean spending less time with friends and family. It may mean jeopardizing my grade in another course.

My goals and priorities determine what I will do; they also determine what I will *not* do. This is the most difficult aspect of being a goal-oriented student. I am forced to admit that although I may be able to do *anything*, I simply cannot do *everything*. The ability to make tough decisions based on goals and priorities is what separates superstudents from so-so students.

4. Who can I count on to help me improve my grade in chemistry?

Me, myself, and I. That's three. Perhaps my instructor, a classmate, my spouse, the lab assistant, or a professional tutor. I will evaluate all possible human resources.

5. How might I sabotage myself so I don't get a better grade?

I might give up without even trying. I might continue to cross my fingers, close my eyes, and hope for the best. I might put off taking action until it is too late. I might rationalize by saying I cannot afford to put more time into chemistry while not admitting that being *unwilling* to pay the price is not the same as being *unable* to pay the price of a higher grade.

By using these five questions, you can establish a plan for achieving any goal: completing a term paper, losing 10 pounds, improving grades, or getting more help around the house. Activating and sticking to the plan takes real backbone.

GOALS TO GO

Goals should be realistic and attainable. Don't become sidetracked by a compulsion for perfection. Some students want not only to graduate but to graduate with honors—or not at all. Settle for pure, unadulterated graduation. Don't take a difficult goal and make it impossible.

Goal-oriented students strive to make everything they do pay off in terms of long-range achievement. They may even take part-time jobs in the health-care industry, thinking they will not only earn needed income but also gain valuable experience.

Instructors advance strong arguments for and against such practice. The "pros" say such jobs provide flexible hours, give students a taste of the real world, boost confidence, and supplement the limited clinical experience provided by the school. The "cons" say such jobs are exhausting and usually pay poorly. The menial jobs offered to students provide meager clinical experience and imprint subordinate status, a mindset that is difficult to break.

Should *you* take a job in the health-care industry? Again, remember that your goal is to graduate. Choose the job that best contributes to that goal.

If you are thoroughly intimidated by the clinical setting, a hospital job may increase your confidence. As your confidence grows, your performance will improve. On the other hand, if you are floundering academically, stop working altogether or look for a low-stress job that allows time for study, such as being a desk clerk, night watchman, or dispatcher. When choosing your job, be practical. The better the salary, the fewer hours you have to work and the more time you can devote to your education.

Stick to business during business hours. Keep your eye focused on the finish line and you will take fewer detours. Keep evaluating each activity and assignment in terms of your goals. For example, is what you are doing at this very moment contributing to one of your goals? YES. Keep reading!

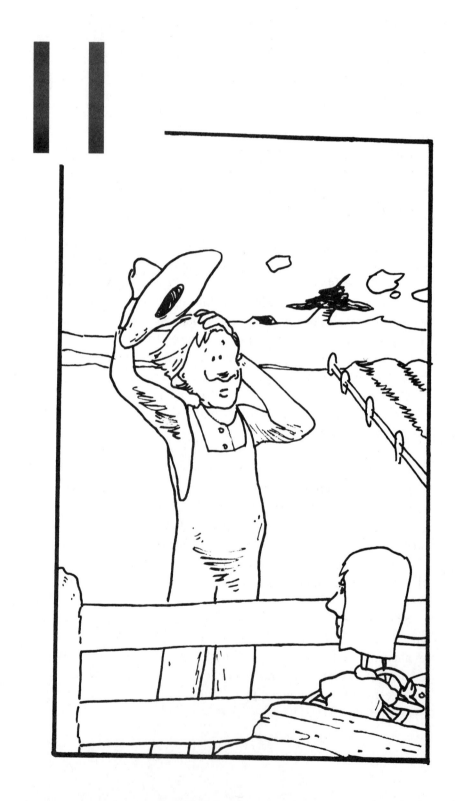

YOU CAN'T GET
THERE FROM HERE

"A problem is nothing but concentrated opportunity."
—Dr. Norman Vincent Peale

After wandering through the New England countryside and becoming hopelessly lost, the motorist stopped and asked a farmer for directions. The farmer paused, then shook his head and replied, "You can't get there from here."

It's an old joke, but the punch line is one that nursing students hear all too often. When you find it necessary to ask for guidance and you are given a you-can't-get-there-from-here answer, don't believe it. Ask again. Ask someone else.

"I wanted to take a business course as an elective, but I didn't have the necessary prerequisite. My advisor suggested I choose something else. Instead, I went to the professor and told him what I hoped to gain from the class and why my life experiences should count as the prerequisite. He granted permission. It was one of the best classes I have ever taken."

Many students make the mistake of asking only one person—often not even the right person. Before you give up, get a second opinion and perhaps a third. Asking for what you want is no guarantee that you will get it, but *not* asking guarantees failure.

59

If you are going to find your way from one end of nursing to the other, make sure you pack plenty of persistence. If one approach doesn't work, switch to another. Be bold enough to deal directly with the people involved and bright enough to bring concrete evidence.

"One of our instructors talked so fast we could not keep up with her. Several of us asked her to slow down, but within a few minutes she would be spewing forth facts and figures at an incomprehensible rate. Our test scores went down. Finally, we decided to record one of her lectures. We made an appointment and played the tape back to her. After listening she apologized and changed her style. Our test scores improved."

Instructors are not mind readers. If you need help, speak up.

"In one of our courses, 10 different teachers presented material. There was some conflicting information, and as the final exam drew closer, we got very worried. Who could we trust for the *correct* answer? We asked *all* the teachers to attend a review session. We asked questions and finally got straight answers."

Faculty members are not purposely insensitive; they are just insanely busy. A major problem for you may look minor on their overcrowded "TO DO" list. Instead of hoping the instructor will deal with your problem quickly, set a definite time. If you say, "I'll check back with you at 4 o'clock tomorrow," you will be less likely to get lost in the shuffle. When you show up the next day, you will either get your answer or reinforce the urgency of your need. It's better to find out that your problem has been overlooked for 24 hours than for 2 weeks.

When meeting a problem head on, a good way to rally support is to draft a petition. Follow proper channels and stick to your guns.

"Our library wasn't open on Sundays. We wrote a petition and virtually everyone signed it. The class officers presented it to the dean.

"We were given all sorts of excuses why it couldn't be done. We just kept pushing for it. Like when we were told the budget wouldn't allow it—all sorts of students volunteered to help staff on a rotating basis.

"Finally, they agreed to open for 4 hours on Sunday afternoons. Traffic in the library has been so heavy they are talking about expanding weekend hours next fall."

Complaining is always easier than generating creative alternatives. Before you call attention to a problem, have several possible solutions in mind. In the following situation the students didn't just let off steam, they proposed a way to streamline the system:

"We were required to write out six full nursing-care plans on our patients. Students were staying up so late and coming to clinical so tired they could not function very well.

"We asked the instructors if we could do some of our care plans orally. We figured you have to know your stuff thoroughly either way. The instructors agreed to a trial period. The new system worked so well that both students and instructors voted to keep it going."

In all five of the above examples the students managed to "get there from here." You can be successful, too—*IF* you have the right kind of drive.

PSYCHOLOGY BEHIND THE WHEEL

By now you have noticed that students have very different driving styles. Some are passive. Some are aggressive.

You can always tell passive drivers by the tread marks on their backs. They are quiet, overly cautious, excessively polite, and indecisive. Always waiting to be told what to do and where to go, they create bottlenecks and are a menace to other drivers as well as to themselves.

Aggressive drivers are fast and reckless. They honk once, and if you don't get out of their way, they run right over you. Their hit-and-run techniques leave the nursing course looking like a demolition derby. They don't care who gets hurt as long as they get where they want to go.

Both passive and aggressive students have low self-esteems. Some have none.

As a student you occupy a subordinate role, and most of us have found that "subordinate" is a euphemism for "inferior." Even though you are not inferior, when you occupy the lesser position, as in parent-child, employer-employee, doctor-nurse, teacher-student, you may begin to have self-doubts. You may feel inferior and behave in inferior ways.

For whatever comfort it is, this problem occurs at all levels of education. Students working on their master's degrees and doctorates experience similar feelings. They begin to question their intelligence and worth. It is just inherent in the role of student.

You don't have to be either passive or aggressive. You can choose a style that is neither reticent nor reckless. You can choose to be *assertive*.

THE ASSERTIVE LANE

Assertiveness is an attitude, coupled with action, that allows you to move through traffic without being injured or injuring others. One way to become more assertive is to adjust your attitude. As your attitude changes, so will your actions.

To offset feelings of inferiority, try viewing your instructors as your employees. After all, you are paying them to teach you the fine art of nursing. They work for you. And, as an employer, you have the right to make requests, ask for improvements, evaluate work performance, and expect loyalty, courtesy, and prompt attention.

An easier way to become more assertive is to adjust your actions. As your behavior changes, so will your attitudes.

How do assertive students act? They stand tall, look you in the eye, and speak up. They are honest enough to express their feelings but tactful enough to protect your dignity. They will laugh with you but never at you. And they love to laugh at themselves.

They are not afraid to say:

"I prefer . . . ."
"I dislike . . . ."
"I am concerned . . . ."
"I need . . . ."
"I want . . . ."
"I do not understand . . . ."

"I disagree . . . ."
"I expect . . . ."

Assertive students are able to accept compliments graciously. They are able to accept criticism thoughtfully. When they fail, they look on failure as a learning experience. Then they adjust their course and head off in a new direction.

When faced with tough problems, they look for solutions instead of scapegoats. They are not interested in plotting to get even—they are too busy planning to get ahead. They are not afraid to make decisions and actively pursue their goals.

Basically, assertive students are realists with optimistic overtones. They share common qualities: positive persistence, boldness, and confidence.

Many nursing schools have integrated assertiveness training into the curriculum. On the surface these skills appear so simple that many overlook the potential power of such a tool. Few appreciate the length of time it takes to become proficient with assertiveness: a lifetime.

Passive and aggressive students may survive the nursing curriculum, but only assertive students have the drive to thrive. The same is true of graduate nurses. Only assertive professionals thrive and consistently manage to "get there from here."

12

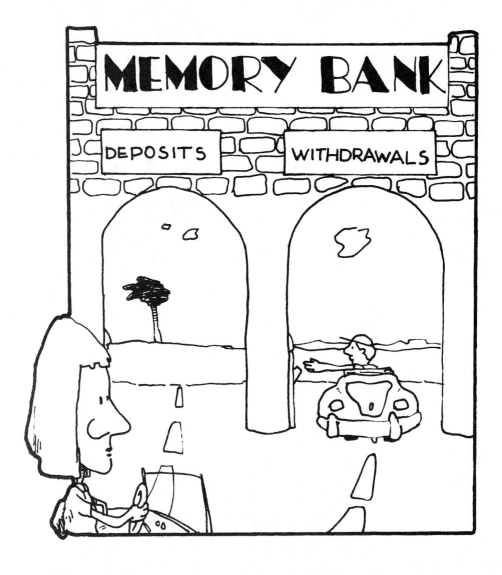

DRIVE-UP TELLER

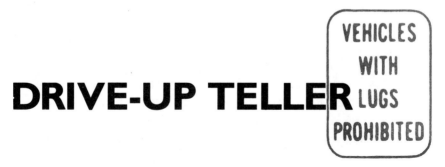

VEHICLES WITH LUGS PROHIBITED

"My memory is so bad, that many times I forget my own name!"

—Cervantes,
Don Quixote

If you are always in a hurry, you probably like the drive-up window at the bank. You can make transactions without even leaving your car. But you still need to fill out the proper forms. You can't just throw money at the drive-up teller and expect it to land in your account.

The same is true of the Memory Bank. You can't just throw information in its general direction and expect to find it later in your account.

The Memory Bank has two branches: short-term and long-term. Cramming is like making a massive deposit in the short-term branch. As long as you withdraw it almost immediately, the lump sum remains intact. If you check on your account a week later, you will find that your deposit has dwindled. A month later you will find a considerable loss. Six months later the account will be closed.

If you want sufficient "funds" available when you go to write state board exams, you cannot rely on your short-term memory bank. The only way to stay solvent is to make deposits in the long-term branch.

The drive-up teller at the long-term branch is best at handling small, regular deposits. Every time you review information, you add to your account. When you review your account, you add interest.

VEHICLES
WITH
LUGS
PROHIBITED

If you tell yourself and others that you have a poor memory, you give your mind permission to forget. Another self-fulfilling prophecy comes true. Instead, tell yourself you have a good or even a great memory. Desire plus confidence pays big dividends.

Some things you think you've forgotten you never actually knew in the first place, such as when you don't quite catch a person's name but you nod and move on.

In the classroom you can't afford to nod and move on. If you don't quite catch the information, ask the instructor to spell the name of the drug or disease. If your notes say there are six common side effects but you can only account for five, ask for the sixth. Get complete, correct information and fix it firmly in your mind.

You cannot remember what you do not understand. One way to check your understanding is to paraphrase the information or think of examples to see whether you really grasp the principles involved.

Information must be meaningful if it is to be remembered. Merging the information with previous or present experiences enables it to be properly catalogued, stored, and retrieved for future use.

When classroom and clinical experiences are synchronized, memory is enhanced. Unfortunately, the two are often out of synch. Only reading about Huntington's chorea simply does not have the same impact as reading about it *while* caring for a patient with the disease.

MEMORYCISE

Experts often compare memory to a muscle that improves with exercise. Stay in shape; work your memory. Experiment with various techniques like visualization and mnemonics.

An example of visualization is picturing yourself paddling a microscopic canoe along the bloodstream. Envision passing through each chamber of the heart and navigating the entire system, down to the smallest capillaries. The more vivid or ludicrous the imagery, the more likely you are to remember.

Mnemonics is another key to opening the memory bank. For example, taking the first letter of each word in a series and forming a new word such as *vibgyor* may help you remember the order of the colors in the rainbow: violet, indigo, blue, green, yellow, orange, and red. Another way to remember a list of items is to make a sentence using the first letter of every word. Two common ones in the health sciences are (1) "On old Olympus' towering top, a Finn and German viewed a hop," and (2) "Never lower tiny perambulator, mamma might come home." The first sentence helps you remember the twelve cranial nerves (olfactory, optic, oculomotor, trochlear, trigeminal, abducens, facial, acoustic, glossopharyngeal, vagus, accessory, hypoglossal), and the second is for the bones of the wrist (navicular, lunate, triangular, pisiform, multiangular/greater, multiangular/lesser, capitate, and hamate).

If you want to amass a wealth of information, the following are two ways to make deposits in the Memory Bank.

I. Listening and Learning

To get the most out of the hours you spend in the classroom, follow these three rules: (1) show up, (2) sit in the front, and (3) look alive! Arrive on time with all necessary equipment. Come rested, nourished, and eager. Choose a seat near the front, away from distractions. Lean forward. Smile. Make eye contact with the instructor. Concentrate. The more you can absorb during class time, the less you will have to absorb on your own time.

Since you are able to hear three times faster than most instructors are able to speak, your mind will have time to wander. Instead of doodling or daydreaming, use that time to organize your notes, differentiate between facts and opinions, fill in gaps, underline material emphasized, and think of practical applications.

During class listen to your inner voice. Are you criticizing the lecturer's ability or appearance? Are you busily refuting or belittling what is being said? When you study under a less-than-ideal instructor, you must make a conscious effort to separate the content from the person presenting it. Avoid running internal arguments or making snide comments to yourself. Listen and learn despite what you think of the instructor.

TAKE NOTES, but don't try to write down every word the instructor says. Few authors and even fewer lecturers are worth quoting verbatim. Before you move your pen, listen. Condense what is said and convert it into your own words. Five minutes of lecture may yield only five words.

Write legibly. Create your own shorthand, but be consistent so that you will be able to decipher it. Here are some abbreviations and symbols that can speed notetaking and thus give you more time for listening.

♀	female
♂	male
>	greater than
<	less than
=	equals, the same
≠	does not equal, different
×	times
→	leads to, going
←	from, away
↑	up, increasing, above
↓	down, decreasing, under
$	dollar
c̄	with
s̄	without
⊕	positive

⊖	negative
Q.	question
A.	answer
q.	every
∴	therefore
∵	because
~	approximately
Hx	history
Dx	diagnosis
Rx	treatment, prescription

Use this space to write or draw other abbreviations and symbols you frequently use. Compare with classmates.

Make your notes fun to read. Use different colors of paper or ink. Toss in an occasional joke or cartoon.

Some students divide their notebook so that the left-hand page contains text notes and the right-hand page contains class notes. Others prefer separate notebooks for readings and lectures. In either case leave generous margins where you can make study lists or insert new material.

After class review your notes as soon as possible. Literally take notes on your notes. Use the margins to summarize. Look for broad principles, see if you understand relationships, separate major from minor facts, assemble any lists worth memorizing, check for discrepancies between lecture and text, and write down questions that occur to you.

II. Reading and Remembering

While reading a journal for nurse educators, an article title caught my eye: "The Relative Influence of Identified Components of Text Anxiety in Baccalaureate Nursing Students." TEXT anxiety? It was a typographical error missed by some proofreader asleep at the switch. The article was on *test* anxiety, not text anxiety.

But I quickly latched onto the idea. If there isn't a disorder called text anxiety, there should be. For example, adult health nursing textbooks average 2000 pages in length. They will soon have to come equipped with wheels because they're too heavy to carry around. Five years ago a dozen consultants would be involved in producing a nursing text. Today as many as five dozen experts contribute to each textbook.

If your nursing books appear to be written in a foreign language, they are. They are written in Latin mixed with technical jargon. Instead of skipping over unfamiliar words, flip to the glossary at the back of the text and keep a medical-nursing dictionary close at hand.

Immerse yourself in the language. Study common root words, suffixes, and prefixes. Make flash cards and carry them with you (see Appendix C).

As you struggle to learn this new language, be acutely aware of your feelings and frustrations. Once you begin speaking "Medicalese" like a native, it is easy to forget what patients and their families go through as they struggle to understand us.

As a nursing student you will have not only a horrendous amount of reading but a horrendous amount of *hard* reading. Educators use a formula based on the length of words and sentences to assess the relative difficulty of written material and assign a grade level to it. For example, the *Reader's Digest* requires grade 8 reading ability, and the *Wall Street Journal* requires grade 10 ability. Nursing students in one baccalaureate program used the formula on their medical-surgical text and found that it required grade 17 ability!

When you need 5 years of college to understand a required freshman text, you realize the importance of reading skills.

If you are a poor reader, you will need help sharpening your skills or else you will not survive the nursing curriculum. Ask about programs to improve reading speed and comprehension. Commercial courses are available, but they are usually expensive. Your school may offer a comparable course for much less and may even give you college credit for it.

Here are some tips to help you get more out of your reading time:

Before you begin reading. Pick a place with no distractions, or if you're in your room, padlock the refrigerator, turn off the TV, disconnect the phone, and hang a DO NOT DISTURB sign on the door. Sit at a desk so you can take notes. Choose a chair that is comfortable but not too comfortable. You don't want to doze off. If you need glasses, wear them, and always make sure you have sufficient light.

Ask yourself *why* you are reading this particular material. Consult the chapter objectives if they're provided. Decide whether your mission is to uncover facts, understand principles, answer specific questions, assess relevance, or create a term paper or a research project of your own.

Before reading the first paragraph, take a couple of moments to SKIM the entire chapter or article. To understand what the author considers important, look at section headings, any bold type, italicized words, illustrations, diagrams, charts, or graphs. Read the whole summary. Examine the study questions provided. To understand what your instructor considers important, check the course outline, objectives, study questions, and any handouts pertaining to this assignment.

While you read. Don't just go through the motions. Remember, it's not what you put into reading, it's what you get out of it that counts. The best way to remember what you read is to TAKE NOTES. A much less effective way is to use a highlighter or to underline as you read. Reading by itself is a poor third choice.

Instruct your mind to focus on the material. Watch for connecting words, qualifiers, and punctuation marks that can completely change the meaning. Reread difficult passages slowly. Move your lips. Reading aloud can increase comprehension.

Read to understand, not to memorize. As you take notes, put the material in your own words. If you can put the material in your own words, you understand it. If you understand it, you can remember it.

Vary your speed. (Average reading speed varies from 100 to 400 words per minute.) One of the quickest ways to improve both speed and comprehension is to use your fingertips to "underline" the sentences as you read. A comfortable position is to turn your palm up and use your middle and index fingers. This action pulls your eyes along the page, enabling you to see more words at a time. It also reduces the chances of losing your place or staring at one word while your mind goes elsewhere.

Maintain a positive attitude. Try to keep an open mind. Resist the urge to argue with the author. If you find statements that seem contradictory or confusing, place a question mark in the margin and ask the instructor for clarification.

After reading. Quickly review your notes or scan what you have underlined in the text. Try to sum up the chapter in your own words. Take a second look at any illustrations, charts, or diagrams. Can you explain them without rereading? Can you answer the author's study questions? Your instructor's study questions?

Parking all this information in your long-term memory requires a chemical change to take place in your brain. Excessive physical or emotional activity immediately after a study session can interfere with this process. Instead of going to a football game or fighting with your spouse, put your book under your pillow and sleep on it.

When you check your statement from the long-term memory bank, you will find that you remember every "first" with remarkable clarity—your first patient, your first injection, your first day in surgery. You are also likely to find any information that startled, surprised, amused, or interested you. And you will have total recall of everything your instructor prefaced with, "You don't have to know this for the test, but . . . ." Bank on it!

13

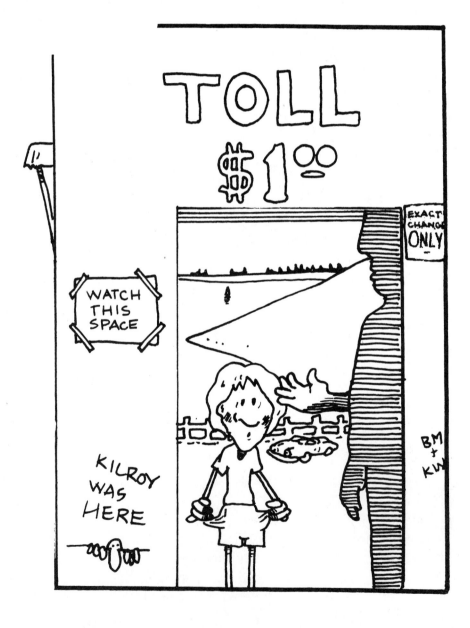

TOLLBOOTH

NARROW BRIDGE

"I have answered three questions, and that is enough."

—Lewis Carroll,
Alice in Wonderland

Zooming along, you spot a tollbooth. The tollgate is down; the red light is flashing. To go from Aspiring Nurse 101 to Aspiring Nurse 202, you have to come up with the correct change: adequate scores on examinations, finished term papers, evidence of clinical competence, and a suitable GPA.

If you search your pockets and come up short, you may be able to persuade the gatekeeper to let you postpone payment. With an INCOMPLETE in hand you are allowed to "pass."

Don't delude yourself into thinking you can easily make up for lost time on the next leg of the course. Each leg is more difficult than the last, and if you are already pushing hard just to keep up, there will be almost no time for making up.

If you are not seriously ill and no one in the family is dying, it is far better to buckle down and complete this term now. Cut out the frills, get a tutor, burn the midnight oil, forget perfection, and accept a grade that is a notch lower than you'd like. Don't try to carry this term's work into next term.

Testing takes a heavy toll on many students. As test time approaches, they experience headaches, dizziness, diarrhea, insomnia, nausea, and assorted muscle cramps. No amount of studying reduces the panic. During the first few moments of the exam they literally lose their minds. Everything goes blank.

"I was a babbling nervous wreck, flapping
around the room like a wild animal,
pouring sweat and unable to concentrate
on any one thought for more than two or
three seconds at a time."
—Hunter S. Thompson,
Fear and Loathing in Las Vegas

Everyone experiences some degree of test anxiety. What may surprise low-performance students is that high-performance students experience the very same physical symptoms, but they instruct their minds not to pay any attention to them. Instead they focus on the test. They quickly become absorbed in the task at hand, and their physical symptoms disappear. High-performers don't worry about *how* they are doing; they concentrate on *what* they are doing.

If you begin to panic during an exam, close your eyes for a moment. Breathe slowly and deeply. Talk positively to yourself. Knock off the easy questions first. This builds confidence and helps you perform to the best of your ability on the remainder of the test.

If you know a student who suffers from such extreme test anxiety that it would be more properly called "test terror," get him or her to professional help.

High-performance students automatically use some simple skills that boost their scores. If you are a student who knows the material as well as your study partners, yet you consistently score lower than they do, these skills can help you even the score.

PREPARATION FOR TESTING

High-performers find out everything they can about the teacher and the test. First, they study the teacher. Is this instructor bent on helping students succeed or on weeding out as many students as possible? Is this a person obsessed with trivia or one who concentrates on principles, ideas, and relationships? What are this person's special interests and areas of expertise?

Second, they gather all the information they can about the test. What kind of test will it be? Multiple-choice or essay? What material will be covered? Text and lecture only, or other reading assignments and laboratory work as well?

The best source of information on the test is the teacher. Just ask! Most are perfectly willing to share this information. You may also find it helpful to ask former students.

An excellent way to prepare for a new test is to study an old one. You may be surprised to learn that many instructors leave copies of their old tests on file at the library or in the department office. Even if the instructor has changed, chances are the course content hasn't. Many questions will be reworded but recognizable.

Believe it or not, you are better off with a teacher who gives frequent tests and quizzes. If there are only two tests given all term, too much is riding on each. By the time you figure out the teacher's style, it is almost too late to improve your grade. If you have a teacher who skimps on tests, it becomes even more important to track down everything possible about the exam beforehand.

When is the best time to begin studying for exams? The first day of class. Successful students attend class religiously, listen intently, take careful notes, and mark information the instructor emphasizes for special study. Soon after each class they condense their notes and review them frequently. (For more study tips see Chapter 9, "More Miles Per Gallon.")

Begin studying for a specific test 2 or 3 weeks in advance. Remember these words: READ * WRITE * REVIEW * RECITE. As you *read, write!* Don't just underline. Jot down the main facts, names, dates, ideas, and relationships. Put everything in your own words. If you can do that, you understand it. If you understand it, you can remember it. *Review* what you've written. Condense your notes. Reread them as often as possible. Close your text or notebook and *recite* what you have learned.

Most students find it helpful to study for tests with a partner or a small group. You often discover things you may have overlooked or underemphasized. When you coach other students, you gain a better grasp of the material yourself.

Some major tests are not given in the regular classroom. Find out where the test will be given. Visit the room and actually spend time studying there. The more comfortable you are in the test room, the more relaxed you will be and the better you will perform.

24 Hours Before the Test

Keep food intake and exercise on the light side. Lay out equipment you want to take with you: pens, pencils, erasers, scratch paper, blue books, calculator, wristwatch, sweater, and, if it is a long test, a snack like M&Ms, peanuts, or raisins.

Surround yourself with pleasant, positive people. Avoid situations that depress or aggravate you.

Ten Minutes Before the Test

Arrive at the test site 10 minutes before the exam. That's enough time to relax and not enough time to panic. Choose a seat away from windows, doors, aisles, friends, and enemies. If you are left-handed, make sure you get a left-handed desk.

Breathe slowly, deeply. Tense and relax your muscles, especially those in your neck and shoulders. Give yourself a pep talk, not an ultimatum.

During the Test

Listen carefully to oral instructions. Ask for clarification if confused. Read written instructions carefully. Take time to work through any sample questions provided. It will save you time in the long run.

Skim the entire test. How many questions are there? How much time can you allow for each? Are the questions weighted differently? For example, 100 multiple-choice questions may be worth only 40 percent of the grade, the matching section worth 10 percent, and the two essay questions worth 50 percent. Divide your time accordingly.

If marking on the test is allowed, scribble things you are afraid you will forget on one of the corners—names, dates, formulas, principles. Circle or underline key words and phrases in the instructions. Examine the stem of each question for significant phrases like "same as," "opposite of," or "only one."

Work quickly. Leave the toughies and time wasters for last. Remember that many answers are found or alluded to in other questions. Keep your eyes open.

A word of caution: since you will be skipping over some questions, periodically check to make sure the number on the question and the number on the answer sheet match.

Tips for MULTIPLE-CHOICE Items

Read directions carefully.

Work quickly. Put a star or checkmark by questions you want to return to later if you have time.

Formulate your own answer before you read the answers given.

Read every given answer.

Eliminate implausible answers.

Watch for absolutes and qualifiers. Answers containing "always," "never," "all," or "none" are usually incorrect.

In many nursing exams multiple-choice questions will be related to rather lengthy case studies. To avoid delays caused by rereading, scan all questions *before* reading the case study. Then your eyes will be more attuned to the important information.

Tips for TRUE-FALSE Items

The longer the T-F statement, the more likely it is to be TRUE.

There are usually more TRUE statements because they are easier to write.

Most statements come verbatim from text or lecture. If it looks familiar, play your hunch.

Statements containing "all," "only," "always," or "because" are usually FALSE.

Statements containing "none," "generally," or "usually" are more often TRUE.

If the statement is long or complicated, break it into smaller parts. Remember, if one part is false, the whole statement is FALSE.

Don't change answers. On T-F items your first impression is usually correct.

Tips for MATCHING Items

Check to see whether answers are used only once or more than once.

Do easy matches first.

Work down the column with the longest phrases.

Look for patterns: dates-events, terms-definitions, people-contributions.

Tips for SHORT ANSWER and FILL-IN-THE-BLANK Items

Look for clues in language and sentence construction.

The length of the blank usually indicates the length of the answer desired.

If you know two possible answers, give both. You will rarely be penalized, and you may get extra credit.

Make an educated guess. Don't leave the blankety-blank blank.

Tips for MATHEMATICAL Items

Read each question very carefully. Write down the givens, what you are expected to find, and any formulas you plan to use.

Estimate the answer before doing calculations so you'll know whether you're close or far afield.

Write legibly, and keep numbers in distinct columns.

Copy accurately.

Check units of measure—ounces, drams, millimeters.

Use a calculator and any other helps permitted.

If abstractions confuse you, substitute simple numbers for symbols.

Check math by working the problem backwards.

If the answer is in multiple-choice form and you haven't the foggiest idea, you can usually eliminate the highest and lowest answers given.

Tips for ESSAY Items

When offered a choice of essay questions, read all of them before deciding which to tackle.

Beside each question, quickly list the facts and ideas that pop into your head.

Budget your time. Spend 50 percent outlining the answer and 50 percent writing it.

Know who will be grading the exam. If it will be scored by a teaching assistant, forgo fancy writing and stuff every name, date, fact, idea, and key phrase you can remember into the answer.

Underline key words in directions. Know precisely what you are to do. For example:

Summarize
Means to give a concise review of the main ideas.

Explain
Means to give the how or why of something.

Illustrate
Means to give effective examples.

Discuss
Means to explain and elaborate.

Define
Means to explain the meaning.

List
Means to give a series of items or ideas without elaborating.

Outline
Means to write only main ideas or facts.

Compare
Means to show similarities.

Contrast
Means to show differences.

Organize your essay: title, topic sentence, main body, and conclusion.

Make a final check for mechanics and spelling if time permits.

If you run out of time, write "I ran out of time. Please accept my outline." You will get partial credit, and you may even get full credit.

Questionable Items

If totally confused, don't panic. Ask the test monitor for clarification.

Don't let toughies derail you. Move on to the next question. Your subconscious mind will go to work on the tough one while your conscious mind works on the next one. Something in another question may jog your memory or clear up confusion.

Break long, complicated questions into small, manageable parts. Read slowly, moving your lips or subvocalizing each word.

If two answers seem correct, choose the more obvious.

If no answer looks correct, choose the most nearly correct answer.

Give the answer the instructor wants. Don't quibble!

Always guess unless there is a penalty for guessing, in which case play the odds.

If you wish to protest an item, see the instructor after the test but before grades are given out.

Just Before Turning in Your Test

Erase all stray marks on the answer sheet.

Check that your name is on each sheet.

Reread directions.

Look at any questions you have flagged for further consideration. If you honestly believe an answer should be changed, change it. You will probably be correct. Just don't waffle back and forth and back again.

Fill in all the blanks.

Use all the time available.

Never give up.

FINAL TOLLBOOTH: STATE BOARD EXAMS

Taking some college courses is like being vaccinated. Once you've given it a shot and passed, you are "immune." Even if you can't remember anything from the course 2 weeks after the final, you never have to take the course again. For courses like that you can cram. In 3 days you can learn everything you need to pass the course, and 3 days later you can forget it all.

Nursing isn't like that. You will not only be required to *remember*, you will be required to *understand* virtually everything from your basic nursing courses. You will be expected to build on that information in more advanced courses, and every day you will apply what you've learned as you care for patients. The study of nursing demands continuous review. There is no way to cram and survive.

Even after you have successfully completed all your schooling, there is still one final exam standing between you and your license to practice nursing. Although everyone reviews for state boards, no one can cram. That's why the best time to begin studying for the state board exams is the first day—and every day—of class.

14

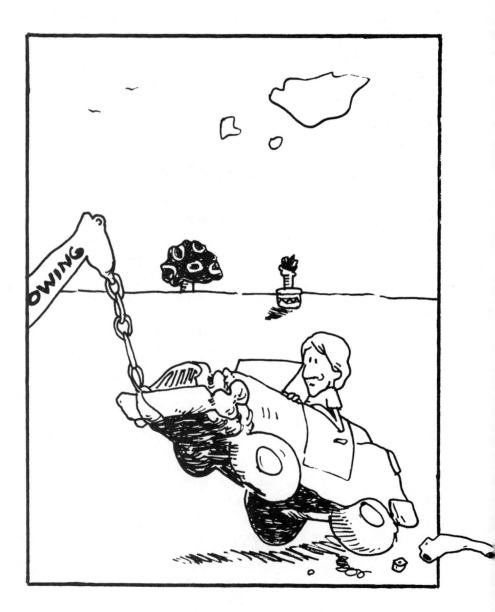

TOTALED

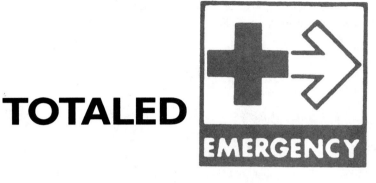

EMERGENCY

"**I** failed! Now I'll never be a nurse!"

Hold on. Before you declare yourself a total wreck, take a closer look at the damage. You may not require a tow truck. You may just need some emergency road service.

If you've flunked an exam, bombed on a term paper, been chewed out by an instructor, or had an irate patient demand to see a "real" nurse, it can be devastating, but it is far from fatal.

Most failures signal a need for change, not an end to all your career aspirations. A poor performance in the classroom or clinical area warns you that things are not going as they should. Heed the warning.

The first step is to determine exactly what happened. Is this an isolated incident or a symptom of an underlying problem? Occasionally failure is due to circumstances beyond your control. *Occasionally*.

To fail has several different meanings. For example, to fail means:

- To lose strength; to fade away or die away; to stop functioning.
- To fall short.
- To become absent or inadequate, to be deficient.
- To disappoint the expectations or trust of someone.

Let's look at how each of these meanings applies to the most common reasons for student failure and explore possible remedies.

"To Lose Strength, to Fade Away or Die Away, to Stop Functioning"

Lack of commitment. This is the Number One reason for failure. Becoming a nurse is not a driving passion. Either you have temporarily lost sight of your goal or you have changed goals—consciously or unconsciously. Your interest is waning. You don't really hate nursing, but you don't really love it. You are lukewarm, and it is beginning to show in your grades.

Remedy: Everyone has a slump now and then. You may need a good night's sleep, a vitamin supplement, a day by the seashore, or a pep talk from a nurse who loves her work. For lingering slumps, talk with your advisor or a guidance counselor. It may be wise to voluntarily step out of school for a while rather than having failure make your exit mandatory.

Laziness. Becoming a nurse is requiring a lot more work than you ever imagined. Frankly, you can't summon up the vim, vigor, and vitality required to keep pace with the rest of the class.

Remedy: Shove it in gear or start looking for a less demanding way to make a living.

Illness. Sudden illness in yourself or a family member can throw a monkey wrench in the best-laid plans. Student nurses are on such an "unforgiving" time schedule that a few days out of commission can spell disaster.

Remedy: If the interruption is brief and you can get up to speed quickly, you may be able to catch up and finish the term successfully. If not, negotiate with the individual instructors for an "Incomplete" or an alternate assignment. Talk with your advisor about all the options. Check on the school's policy regarding withdrawal without penalty. Before you take the off ramp, make sure there is an on ramp available. Once off the track, you may be out of the course for a year or more.

"To Fall Short"

Lack of ability. Caring *about* sick people is one thing; caring *for* them is quite another. Nursing demands peak performance physically, mentally, and emotionally. You may be intellectually gifted but a basket case emotionally. You may be emotionally strong but physically frail. Not everyone has the right mix of talents, skills, and abilities to make a success of nursing.

Remedy: Determine which limitation is causing the failure. You can shore up sagging abilities, but it may require an inordinate amount of time and energy. Decide whether you are both willing and able to take the corrective action. Seek professional counsel.

Self-defeating behaviors. This might be more accurately called "imagined lack of ability." If you expect to fail, you will rarely be disappointed. Pessimists, nitpickers, worrywarts, perfectionists, and procrastinators are some who fit into this category.

Remedy: Sometimes just recognizing a self-defeating behavior can change its impact so dramatically that you can convert failure into success. Other times these behaviors are so entrenched that professional help is required to overcome their crippling effects.

"To Become Absent or Inadequate, to be Deficient"

Absenteeism. When Woody Allen was asked the secret of his success, he quipped that showing up was 80 percent. Students who fail, fail to show up for class. Grades are directly correlated with class attendance.

Remedy: Force yourself to attend every class. Sit near the front.

Poor study habits. College students have to run full speed just to keep up. If your study skills are not up to snuff, your workload will be doubled. Not only will you have to master the subject matter, you will have to master study skills as well. By the time you realize the importance of being efficient and effective in your study habits, it may be too late. The damage will be done.

Remedy: *Habit* is the key word. Habitual study. Consistently putting in time with the books is vital if you are to survive. Knowing how to get the most out of your study time will help you thrive. For extra help, see Chapters 9, 12, 13, and 20.

Outside activities. Although outside activities can greatly enrich your life, an overdose can kill you. The famous last words of many former students who failed to graduate are, "Never let school interfere with your education."

You may be a first-time-away-from-home student who is intoxicated by your new freedom. You are so busy experiencing life that you haven't had time to think about grades. Or you may be Superstudent, who edits the school paper, serves as council president, builds the homecoming float, and works 20 hours a week as a clerk. Or you may be the midlife mother-wife, promising that nothing will change just because you've added studenting to your already busy schedule. You still manage to keep the house spotless, teach Sunday school, manage the charity bazaar, and turn out gourmet meals when entertaining.

The only thing wrong with outside activities is that they gobble up time, and time is an irreplaceable resource. An A in homecoming, parenting, or partying will not balance an F in anatomy, microbiology, or organic chemistry.

Remedy: Recognize that to succeed as a student you will have to limit outside activities for a few years. Reevaluate the people, events, and things in your life. Simplify, simplify, simplify. Keep a couple of the most satisfying, and slough off everything else.

"To Disappoint the Expectations or Trust of Someone"

Perhaps the most difficult aspect of failure is having to face all those people who expected you to become a nurse. Your parent or spouse says, "I don't understand. Why are you dropping out? You've wanted to be a nurse since you were 6 years old."

What do you say to people like that? First, remind them that you aren't 6 years old anymore, and suggest that no one should be bound by career choices made in childhood. "Yes, I always dreamed of being a nurse, but now I'm awake. And when I looked at nursing with my eyes wide open, I realized it wasn't the career for me."

Some things are more attractive from a distance, such as a beautiful suit that catches your eye from clear across the store. It looks great on the hanger, but when you try it on it just doesn't fit.

You've tried on nursing. It doesn't fit. Minor alterations are always possible, but major alterations may be impossible—or at the very least, impractical.

Remedy: Whether you failed nursing or nursing failed you, give yourself time to grieve. Loss is always painful, even if it is only a dream that has died. Then get out and shop around for a career that does fit. Someday when you are a successful lawyer, architect, teacher, mechanic, musician, or florist, a nurse will walk by and you'll say with a sigh, "There but for the grace of God (and a few lousy grades) go I."

• • •

A nursing professor is currently serving on a board of directors with a former student whom she failed in a leadership course years before. In retrospect the professor attributes the failure to her own inexperience as a teacher at the time and the student's nonconformity, which was misinterpreted by the faculty.

Today that former student is not only a nurse but heads a multimillion dollar company. And she failed LEADERSHIP!

Neither has mentioned the incident, and frankly, it is driving the professor nuts. I suggested she take her former student to lunch and have a good laugh over it. That failure may have been the catalyst that drove the student to success. After all, the best revenge is living well.

> "Defeat may serve as well as victory to shake the soul and let the glory out."
> —Senator Sam J. Ervin, Jr.

15

HOW TO JUMP-START YOUR BATTERY

"The tougher you are on yourself, the easier life will be on you."
—Zig Ziglar

Have you ever jumped into your car and found the battery dead as a doornail? If you were parked on a hill, you may have tried this simple trick: you let the car start rolling, popped the clutch, and the engine leaped to life.

Sometimes you jump into a term paper and find it dead as a doornail. You sit at the typewriter, fingers poised, but nothing happens. The words won't come.

Instead of sitting immobilized for lack of the *right* words, type *any* words: random thoughts, sentence fragments, even gibberish. Don't waste time agonizing over the opening paragraph; skip to the middle section. Begin anywhere you can. Get rolling, pop the clutch, and your engine will leap to life. Remember, it is easier to steer a moving vehicle, and it is easier to edit than to write.

Have you ever found yourself reading the same sentence for the third time? That's a sure sign your battery is dead. You need to recharge before you continue. Get up and splash some cool water on your face. Stretch. Reach for the ceiling, then bend over and touch your toes. Do a dozen jumping jacks. Then sit down and begin reading again.

Does this sound familiar? "I know I *should* work on my care plan, but I just don't *feel* like it right now." Forget feelings. MOVE! Put the machinery in motion, and the *feeling* will follow.

If you are sitting idle alongside the road, here is one way to jump-start your battery. Take your kitchen timer and set it for 5 minutes. Pick up that required reading, your research notes, or the care plan you have to do, and agree to work on it for just 5 minutes. You can stand anything for 5 minutes, right?

In that few moments something miraculous usually happens. The most inert students are energized. When the timer rings, odds are you will continue the activity. You won't even want to quit.

Another way to conquer procrastination is to make an appointment with yourself. Select a definite day, time, and place to begin working on a project. Keep that appointment.

THE PSYCHOLOGY OF PUTTING IT OFF

Almost every student procrastinates. Some do it because they are rebellious. They hate being told what to do and when to do it. By refusing to meet deadlines, they experience a temporary high and a fleeting feeling of being in charge.

Others are thrill seekers. They see the deadline as the edge of a cliff. Driving pell-mell, they see how close they can come to the edge before chickening out. At the last minute, they veer off and hurriedly do the project.

Some students love to experiment. They want to see whether the instructor really means *DEAD*line or whether special privileges will be granted to keep them from a fatal plunge.

Still others use procrastination to protect their fragile egos. Endorsing the "I-work-better-under-pressure" theory, they try to cram 2 weeks of work into 2 days. In the last few hours they exert superhuman effort. If the project fares well, it affirms their better-under-pressure theory. If the project fares poorly, they comfort themselves with the thought that they *could* have done better. There just wasn't enough time.

Afraid to really put their ability to the test, they continue to procrastinate. After all, wouldn't it be mortifying to work all term and produce only a mediocre project?

OUT OF NEUTRAL AND INTO GEAR

If you are struggling to overcome procrastination, here is another gimmick to help you get moving. Take a piece of paper and fold it in half. On the right-hand side list everything you have to gain by completing a project on time or ahead of schedule. On the left-hand side list everything you have to gain by putting the project off until the last possible moment.

If you are honest, you will have to admit that the only things gained by procrastination are anxiety, guilt, low grades, and other assorted headaches. If you tackle projects promptly and aim for early completion, your grades will rise along with your self-confidence and self-esteem. You will experience relief, joy, a sense of accomplishment, and a certain amount of smugness. You will be able to take time off for good behavior and really enjoy yourself.

Time off is one thing procrastinators actually don't have. Undone work, unmet deadlines, and the dread of facing irate instructors haunt their leisure hours. Every time they pass the library or glance at their dusty typewriters they suffer pangs of guilt. Constantly nagged by the thought of what they *should* be doing, they find it almost impossible to relax.

If you are a particularly stubborn procrastinator, you may have to use the carrot-and-stick approach. This method moves stubborn students as well as stubborn mules. For example, to get students moving, instructors dangle "carrots" like smiles, praise, recognition, good grades, merit scholarships, a spot on the dean's list, and opportunities for choice assignments. For "sticks" they use frowns, criticism, harassment, low grades, probation, and failure.

Some students respond more quickly to carrots, others to sticks. How about you?

To get yourself moving, you can devise your own system of rewards and punishments. When you keep regular study

SEND
HELP

hours or perform assignments promptly, reward yourself. Take a bubble bath, have lunch with a friend, watch your favorite TV program, have a cup of gourmet coffee, read the next chapter in a trashy novel. If you fail to keep regular study hours or to meet a deadline, punish yourself. Take a cold shower, unplug the TV set, go without coffee, contribute money to an organization you despise, eat a bologna-banana sandwich.

To be most effective, your reward and punishment system must be highly individualized. One student's reward is another's punishment. Create your own list (see p. 95).

Just like this list, batteries have both positive and negative poles. Whenever you need a jump-start, use one of your carrots, one of your sticks, or a combination of the two.

Check your battery frequently. If you begin to feel run down, recharge by taking a different route home, eating supper at breakfast time, sending yourself roses, watching a vintage movie, wading in a brook, or diving into a new adventure.

Don't forget that batteries also run down when you turn off your engine but leave your lights on. Turn off your lights. Get some sleep.

CARROTS

People, places, things,
and activities I enjoy

STICKS

People, places, things,
and activities I dislike

16

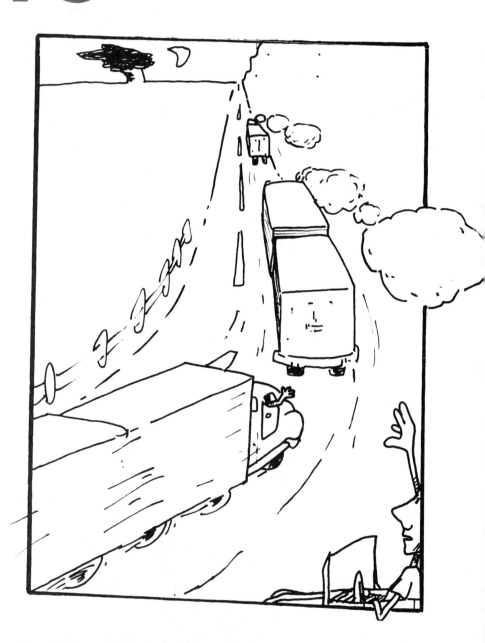

10-4 GOOD BUDDY

"All for one, one for all, that is our device."
—Alexandre Dumas,
The Three Musketeers

Long, lonely stretches of road loom between you and graduation. No one can possibly know the trials and tribulations you are going through. No one except *another nursing student.* That's why the best way to keep on truckin' is to form a convoy.

In a project sponsored by the University of San Francisco to help retain freshman nursing students, faculty members were surprised to learn how much homesickness was a factor in a student's decision to leave school. The first couple of months are the hardest. This is especially true for students who can't get home on weekends because of time, distance, or money problems. To curb the impact of homesickness, the project members suggested linking lonely students together, sponsoring group activities on weekends, or having a local student invite a stranded student home with them. Just letting the homesick students know what they were feeling was normal and temporary helped a lot.

Some of their other suggestions to help freshman nursing students survive included having group and individual counseling sessions; having an intensive orientation program to help students sharpen their study skills and time management abilities; getting the new students involved with upperclassmen in the nursing school; encouraging participation in fun activities as well as study groups; and assisting them with personal problems as well as academic difficulties.*

Nursing students often band together to survive. Without the buddy system, many simply would not make it. When you have to drive in the dark as much as nursing students do, it's reassuring to hear a friendly voice and know you are not alone. Even though you know you must haul your own load, the trip is safer and more enjoyable when you share the road with others.

Safety in Numbers

Traveling with a group reassures you that you are on the right road. Just knowing you are not alone keeps panic at a manageable level. As you exchange ideas and experiences, your confidence grows.

The group helps you clear up mysteries, distinguish facts from rumors, set priorities, and achieve goals. Good buddies not only cheer you up when you are losing, they cheer you on when you are winning.

Belonging to a group has several other advantages:

Working together facilitates problem solving.

"I am in a support group consisting of older students with children. We were all frantically trying to keep our stress levels down and our time-management skills up. After we formed the group, we found we could help each other solve problems on the home front as well as in the classroom. We encourage each other to take 1 day at a time, to prioritize, to do only what needs to be done, and not to hesitate to ask for help—at home or in school."

Camaraderie replaces competition.

"Joining a study group was the best thing I ever did. I learned to compete with myself, not with other students."

Group membership fosters cooperation.

---

*From Cameron-Buccheri R and Trygstad L: Retaining freshman students. Nursing Health Care 10(7):389–393, Sept 1989.

"Instead of every student carrying a whole satchel of books to the clinical area, each student in our group carries a different one. That way all of our books are available for reference, but no one gets a broken back. Besides, there's not enough room in the clinical area to store any more of those 40-pound books!"

Studying with a group means less chance of overlooking or missing important material.

"Our instructors all talk so fast that I knew I was missing things that were important. In study group I spend a few moments comparing my notes with classmates. That way I can fill in the blank spots. My grades have really improved since I started studying with a group."

Strength in Numbers

If you're on your own, you may hesitate to challenge a school policy, call the instructor's attention to inconsistencies, or make special requests. Group support can give you courage.

"We were faced with so much material for each test that we were overwhelmed. We approached the instructors and told them we wanted to have four tests instead of two. And they went for it!"

Studying with friends can lift not only your spirits, but also your GPA.

"I was disappointed in my grade in micro. I thought I had a 'B' going for me, but I received a 'C.' When I mentioned it in my study group, they insisted I talk with the instructor and report back. I did get a 'B'! (There was a computer error.) Without group support and encouragement, I would never have approached the instructor."

Groups can decrease depression and increase productivity.

"Our class was always bitching and complaining about the heavy workload, the tedious assignments, etc. Some of us decided to form a study group with one rule: 'No Bitching.' Instead of complaining about tiresome assignments, we figure out ways to do them better and faster than if we tried to do them alone. We make lists, cross out days on the calendar, and generally encourage each other to think positively. Things still aren't perfect, but we're a lot less depressed."

If you aren't already in a study group, shop around for one. If you can't find one, start one. If you're hesitant, just try it out and see how you like it. For example, organize a temporary group to prepare for one event, such as a major exam or a massive project. If you like studying and working together, you can meet on a more permanent basis.

Your schedule is most likely to mesh with those of other students in your clinical rotation. See if you can interest a half dozen of them in joining you.

Successful study groups have certain ground rules. For the group to be effective, every nursing student in it must agree to the following:

1. Understand and accept the group purpose or mission.
2. Contribute ideas, information, opinions, and feelings.
3. Invite and encourage other members to do the same.
4. Listen intently.
5. Demonstrate respect and support for other members.
6. Help keep the discussion relevant.
7. Periodically help summarize the major points.
8. Give examples and share pertinent clinical experiences.
9. Recognize conflict and controversy as potentially positive, and refuse to see it as a personal rejection.
10. Refrain from eating, smoking, or *knitting* during the session.

How to Make a Good Study Group Better

Time
Always meet at the same time.

Place
Always meet at the same place.

Begin
Always begin on time.

Monitor
Appoint a monitor to keep the group on target and the discussion moving. Focus on the here and now. Don't let the group spend too much time dwelling in the past or fretting about the future.

Goal
At the beginning of the session, state the goal. "Today we will discuss Chapters 4 and 5," or "This group is reviewing for the anatomy midterm."

Discuss
Allow free-flowing discussion of anything relevant to the group's goal. Identify major concepts, clarify discrepancies between text and lecture, share examples from clinical experience, relate theory to practice. If questions arise that cannot be quickly and accurately answered, don't waste time pooling ignorance. Appoint one member to check with the instructor and report back to the group.

Review
Review lecture notes, highlights of outside readings, films, class objectives, lists to be memorized, etc.

Quiz
Drill each other. Use test questions at the end of the chapter or, better yet, construct your own.

"Lately we've each been bringing two 'trivia' questions to group. It's not only fun, it also forces each member to read and review before the study session. Constructing questions has helped me think the way instructors think when they're making up tests."

Summarize
Periodically pause and recap the major points under discussion. At the end of the session, summarize what you have accomplished and list the things that still need to be done.

Divide
Whenever possible, divide tasks and activities.

"We split up the objectives, with each member being responsible for just a few. That person gathers the information and brings copies for everyone to the next meeting. It saves so much time!"

Assign
Assign individuals or subgroups to tasks, and be sure to specify dates for completion.

End
Always end on time.

Socialize
After the official end of the group, members may feel free to leave or to stay and chat. The benefits of playing together should not be underestimated.

"We had a problem maintaining student morale, so about once a month we have some kind of a get-together where we can relax and talk or joke about our problems. Last semester we had 3 hours between classes, and every so often we'd order pizza to be brought in or we'd go out for lunch. At our Christmas party we all got together and composed a letter to Santa telling him about all our 'goofs' in clinical. It was fun and reassuring to hear that everyone else made 'goofs' like I did."

When students form study groups or support groups, they are "networking." You may be interested to learn that student networks reach far beyond your own campus. They operate on a national and an international level. If you would like to extend your network, write to:

National Student Nurses' Association
555 West 57th Street
New York, New York 10019
(212) 581-2211

or

Canadian University Nursing Students' Association
School of Nursing
Université de Montréal
C.P. 6128
Montréal, Québec, Canada
H3T 1J4
(514) 343-6437

Registered nurses band together in groups for the same reason students do—to survive. And for one even better reason—to thrive! If you would like more information about networks available for registered nurses, see Appendixes F and G for the names and addresses of major nursing associations.

Students helping students. Nurses helping nurses. That's a 10-4, Good Buddy.

17

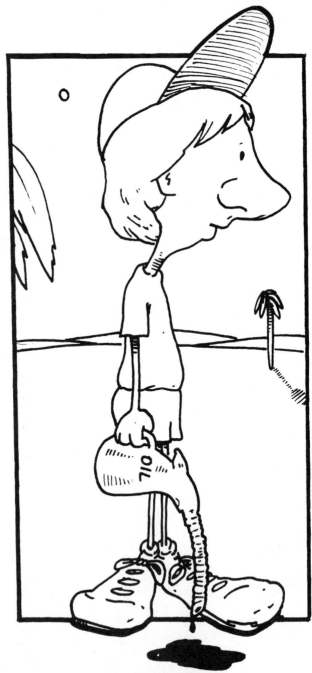

PREVENTIVE
MAINTENANCE

"Fatigue makes cowards of us all."
—Vince Lombardi

If you are a smart driver, you know the value of preventive maintenance. You take simple actions to stop problems before they start. You know that by investing a few minutes, you can add years to the life of your car.

When you stop for gasoline, you automatically check the oil and water. Every few thousand miles you replace the points and spark plugs, examine the fan belt for wear, and grease the joints.

SELF-SERVICE

In fact, you may take better care of your car than you do of yourself. Those of us attracted to the helping professions are often good at taking care of everyone's needs but our own. We talk a lot about high-level wellness, stress management, and self-actualization, but few of us apply those concepts to our own lives.

We wouldn't run our machinery into the ground, but our personal motto seems to be "Don't Stop Till You Drop." We don't even take time to fuel properly. We skip breakfast, eat lunch out of a vending machine, and drive through "Burgers R Us" for dinner.

Isn't it a pity that nursing students don't come equipped with instrument panels? Then you would know at a glance if your engine was overheating or your brake fluid was running low. Unfortunately, you have no gauges, bells, whistles, or warning lights. Before realizing it, you may drive yourself right into a breakdown.

Preventive maintenance for humans is not as clear-cut as it is for vehicles. It probably includes things such as the following:

- Exercising regularly
- Reducing caffeine
- Avoiding unproductive stress
- Eliminating tobacco
- Getting sufficient rest
- Taking vitamin supplements
- Keeping your sense of humor

The key words for a healthy lifestyle are *balance* and *moderation.*

When you find yourself under a lot of pressure and you need to talk things out, you may not be able to find a sympathetic ear. Instead of mumbling to yourself, you may find it helpful to keep a written journal, a daily diary of everything that happens to you as a nursing student. For some reason, talking to yourself on paper is considered sophisticated. Talking to yourself out loud is considered schizophrenic.

Writing allows you to vent feelings safely, unscramble puzzling situations, explore new insights, and put events in perspective. Like a good friend, the journal "remembers" everything you've been through: all the firsts, all the good times, all the adventures and misadventures. On a bad day, when you forget how far you've come, the journal reminds you of your triumphs, not just your tragedies. The journal documents your growth. It chronicles not only your life and times but also the times of your life.

You can purchase an elegantly bound book full of blank pages or use a loose-leaf binder and ordinary notepaper. The journal is for your eyes only. There is no need to worry about spelling, punctuation, or grammar. You may worry about those things later if you decide to convert it into a best-seller.

Being a nursing student can throw everything out of kilter. So pamper yourself. Have regular checkups. Use common sense . . . and WEAR SUPPORT HOSE! Remember, it is easier to prevent problems than to correct them.

18

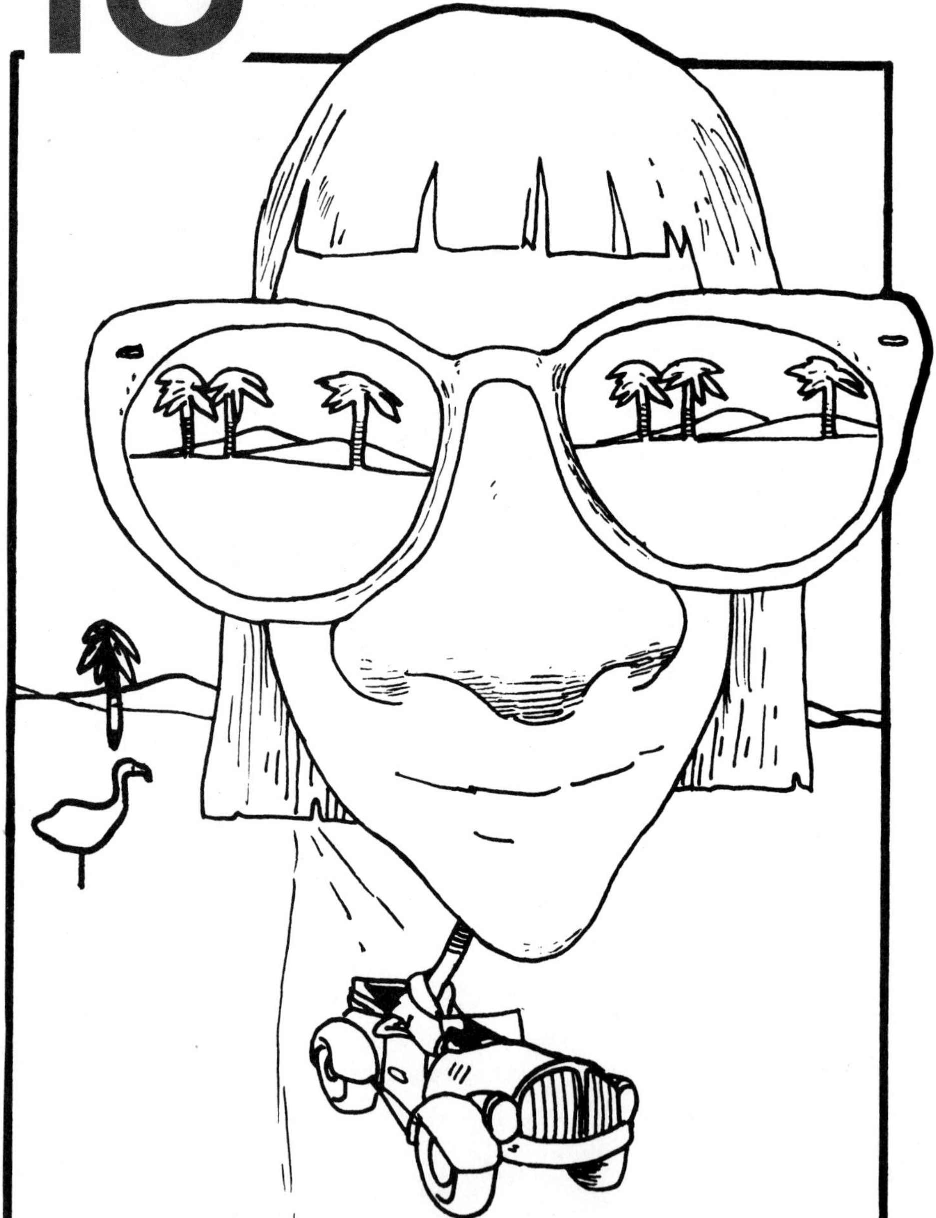

SCENIC ROUTES

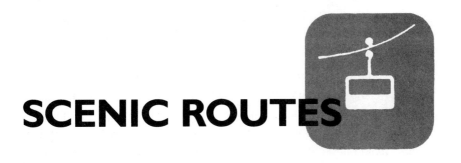

"A university must give its priority to the numerically small but historically significant band of men and women who believe the worth and dignity of knowledge does not depend solely upon its current usefulness."
—Kingman Brewster

As a nursing student you are usually compelled to go for speed and distance. The only chance you have to leave the main highway is through an occasional elective.

When it comes to choosing an elective, be sure to take the scenic route. Get as far away from nursing as possible. A brief excursion to some out-of-the-way discipline can be thoroughly refreshing and can help you return to the hard, fast pace of nursing with renewed energy and unusual insights.

Watch out for what former University of Rochester President Dennis O'Brien calls the "careerist syndrome." Having a rigid, narrow focus on career goals means missing exciting educational opportunities and graduating ill-equipped to deal with a fast-changing, increasingly complex world.

Once in awhile you need a reminder that the whole world does not revolve around science or sickness. There are other worlds: art, music, drama, politics, economics, business, architecture . . . agriculture! Use your electives for field trips to these other worlds.

Nursing requires you to be so perfect and so practical that you may need an elective that allows you to be imperfect and impractical. Use electives for mental-health breaks.

Because advisors are paid to look out for your future, they sometimes overlook your present. Consider your advisor's list of should-and-ought electives, then make your own choice. Instead of choosing an elective that will "expedite things in graduate school," choose one that will help you survive undergraduate school. Trust your instincts. You may be smarter to pass up intermediate statistics and opt for art appreciation.

If you have difficulty persuading your advisors to let you take offbeat electives, remind them that art, music, and drama all have therapeutic applications. Call on their interests in the legal, ethical, economic, or political ramifications of health care. Convince them that public relations is currently receiving as much attention from the hospital hierarchy as patient care. Confess that you have international (or even interplanetary) aspirations for nursing.

If all else fails, produce this ad, which appeared in a big-city newspaper:

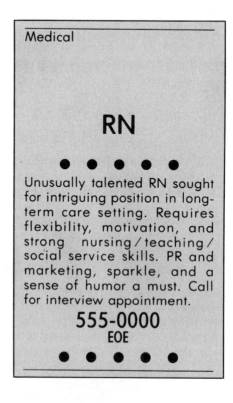

Medical

RN

● ● ● ● ●

Unusually talented RN sought for intriguing position in long-term care setting. Requires flexibility, motivation, and strong nursing/teaching/social service skills. PR and marketing, sparkle, and a sense of humor a must. Call for interview appointment.

555-0000
EOE

● ● ● ● ●

Tell them that this is the job of your dreams and that you need this particular elective to improve your "sparkle" and "sense of humor." Sometimes an elective, just like this classified ad, brings much-needed comic relief. This ad shows that *no* elective should be deemed inappropriate.

Use the entire college catalog when searching for electives. Be brave. Boldly go where no nursing student has gone before. Explore! Enjoy!

19

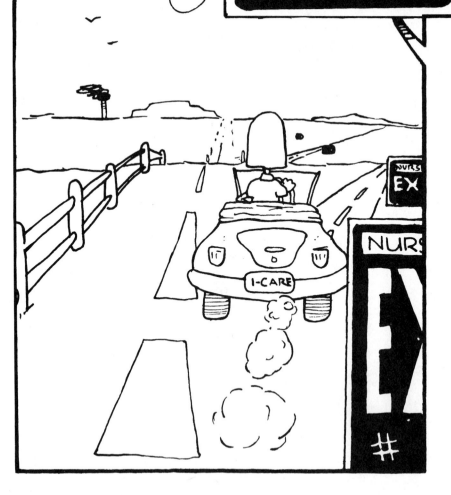

ALTERNATE ROUTES

"Make it thy business to know thyself,
which is the most difficult lesson in the
world."

—Cervantes,
Don Quixote

As you approach nursing, you may be surprised by the number of alternate routes available. Some nurses get off on caring for children, others on caring for the elderly. Some get off on the emergency room, others on intensive care, obstetrics, orthopedics, gastroenterology, or hospice nursing. If you get off on delving into the subconscious, take the exit marked "Psychiatric Nursing." If you prefer the *un*conscious, take the "Operating Room" exit. You may veer off toward school nursing, occupational health nursing, or even private practice. The number of alternate routes will both delight and confuse you.

How do you know which route will be right for you? While in school, you will have several chances to sample alternate routes. Take full advantage of this opportunity. Push yourself to explore as many alternatives as possible.

When I taught at the University of Wisconsin-Madison, clinical experience in psychiatric nursing was an option, not a requirement. The students I had in this class were exceptional. Did they sign up because they thought they had an affinity for psychiatric nursing? No. Most of them were scared. They didn't *have* to come, and many confessed they didn't *want* to come, but they *chose* to come rather than miss a unique opportunity. All were glad they made the trip, even though only a few went on to become psychiatric nurses.

GET OUT AND PUSH

Instead of looking for an easy out or sliding along the path of least resistance, challenge yourself. Cultivate your adventurous streak. To increase your flexibility and tolerance, exercise. Stretch yourself to the limits. You don't have to abandon your goals or values, but you do need to test them. Examine their origins, their accuracy, and their usefulness.

When you hit the open road to nursing, the best thing you can bring along is an open mind. You will be caring for, and working with, people of every race, religion, creed, culture, sex, age, education, and income bracket. Tolerance and flexibility mean survival.

Nurses are supposed to be nonjudgmental—a noble concept that is impossible to attain. You *will* be judgmental. You will judge everyone on the basis of your standards, just as I will judge everyone on the basis of mine.

To keep judgmental attitudes from interfering with professional performance, you have to know yourself inside and out. Take a few moments to describe yourself by answering these questions:

Age?
Sex?
Race?
Ethnic background?
Region of country?
Urban or rural?
Fat or thin?
Religion? How religious?
Political preference? How political?
Education?
Income level?

Pet peeves?
Favorite charities?
Energy level?
Optimistic or pessimistic?
Shy or bold?
Recreational pastimes or hobbies?
Dreams?
Fears?
Family commitments?
Et cetera?

The more answers you have in common with someone, the more comfortable you will be with that person. Unfortunately, you cannot choose your patients or classmates as you do your friends. You have to take what you get and then work at establishing a relationship. The operative word is *work*.

On the highway there is always a right side and a wrong side of the road. In nursing, as in life, the distinctions are not that clear-cut. Every day you will deal with sensitive people and emotionally charged issues. You need to be fully aware of your attitudes on abortion, euthanasia, pain control, venereal disease, suicide, disability, disfigurement, abuse, addiction, and the right to die—to name only a few.

When you find yourself holding views diametrically opposed to those of your patients, classmates, teachers, or coworkers, it is difficult to keep from being offended or from offending others. Knowing your feelings is crucial because attitudes guide actions.

In nursing you need to be able to tolerate a great deal of ambiguity. You have to learn to live with choices that are not yours to make.

Strive to recognize differences as differences. Steer clear of the impulse to label them as right or wrong. You can't live happily in nursing until you understand that your way is only *one way*. There will always be alternate routes.

20

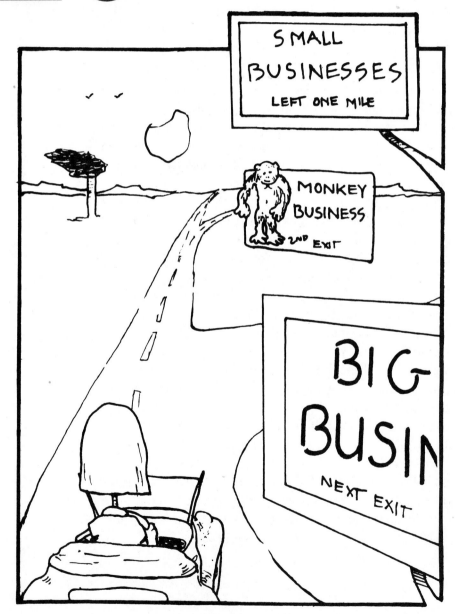

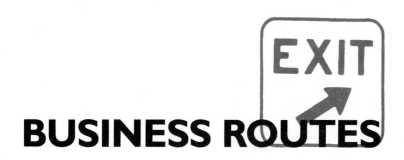

BUSINESS ROUTES

"Words are all we have."
—Samuel Beckett

When you are a student, your business is to deliver words on demand. Whether drafting a term paper, giving a report to the next shift, persuading an instructor to modify an assignment, writing a care plan, presenting an award, making a report to classmates, teaching a patient self-care, or addressing an international meeting, it all boils down to words.

When you need to get down to business, there are two routes you can follow. You can either deliver words in person, or you can deliver words on paper.

WORDS DELIVERED IN PERSON

When you have to deliver words in person, the first rule is *know your audience.* Will there be one person or one hundred? Regular people or professionals? Male or female? Age? Education? Primary interests? Familiarity with the subject? The better you know your audience, the better your chances for a successful presentation.

Next, you have to know the *purpose* of your presentation. Are you supposed to stimulate interest, provide information, arouse to action, teach a skill, or entertain?

Consider how much time you have for your presentation. The amount of preparation time required for a good presentation is inversely proportional to the amount of time allotted. That means it takes more preparation time to give a good 10-minute talk than a good 60-minute talk. The less time you have to deliver, the more efficiently focused, tightly organized, and highly polished you have to be.

When you try to tell your audience "everything," they usually leave with nothing. Good presenters know how important it is to define and limit content.

To prioritize content, ask yourself, "If the audience could take away only *one* idea or piece of information, what should it be?" That becomes your first and foremost objective. What is the second most important idea for them to grasp? The third?

By prioritizing your content, you will know how much time and attention to devote to each section. And if you are allotted less time for your presentation than expected, you will know where to trim it without doing major damage.

The Construction

Taking the three vital objectives you have identified, draft a bare-bones outline. Do whatever reading, research, or interviewing is necessary to flesh it out.

Some students prefer to write out their speeches word for word. That is fine if you promise not to *read* it word for word. Never, ever read your speech. You will bore people to death. Never, ever memorize your speech. You will bore yourself to death.

After you've constructed a comprehensive outline or drafted your entire speech, grab a couple of index cards. Now: reduce your entire speech to a dozen key words or phrases.

The Rehearsal

Pick up your index cards and begin rehearsing. Play with alternate words and phrases. Then, when you stand before the audience, you will not suffer a loss for words or panic when you cannot remember the exact words.

Using a tape recorder during rehearsal is an excellent idea. Listening to yourself for the first time is often a shock. It may not sound like you to you, but that is the way you sound to others. Listen to your voice. Is it lively, well-modulated, clear? Do you mumble, stammer, say "you know" 539 times? Check the pacing and your choice of words.

Resist the compulsion to fill every second with words like "ah . . . uh . . . ahummm." Clearing your throat and coughing are usually nervous attempts to fill empty spaces. Actually, pauses and silences can have a powerful impact. With practice, you can learn to be comfortably quiet between thoughts.

Choose words that are positive. Make no apologies or excuses such as "I wish I had had more time to prepare . . ." or "You probably know more about this subject than I do . . ."

Do not talk down to your audience. Do not snow them with statistics or use half your time dropping names of experts. Steer clear of slang, jargon, and profanity.

Consciously curb nervous gestures like twisting your hair, pulling your ears, blinking rapidly, giggling, playing with your notes, or jingling the change in your pocket.

Sometimes it helps to rehearse in front of a mirror. Then you can see yourself as others see you. This shock may be even greater than that from listening to yourself on the tape recorder. But if you are serious about improving your speaking skills, you have to be willing to critique yourself. Poise will come with practice.

When you rehearse, go through your entire speech from start to finish. If you make a mistake or forget an important point, make a graceful recovery and keep going. You won't be able to start over from the top when you face a live audience.

You also need to time yourself during rehearsal. Inexperienced speakers invariably underestimate the amount of time it takes for delivery. With 2 minutes left, half of their content remains untouched. Remember, nothing makes an audience happier than a speaker who ends on time, unless it is a speaker who ends 5 minutes early.

Have a full dress rehearsal, especially if you plan to wear new clothes or shoes. Test drive your outfit so you know your shoes won't pinch, your skirt won't ride up, and you can reach the top of the chalkboard without splitting a seam. Choose something that is comfortable yet attractive and very professional looking.

Are you a little nervous about your presentation? Good. A bit of anxiety gets the adrenaline flowing and helps you do your best. An overdose of anxiety, however, can paralyze you.

The Countdown

There are several things you can do to keep anxiety under control. For example, visit the room where you will give your presentation. Check out the lighting, acoustics, exits, seating arrangements . . . the nearest bathroom. Stand behind the lectern. Run through a few lines. Decide where you will place any equipment or props. Practice using projectors or other mechanical devices.

If possible, mingle with the audience before your session begins. Introduce yourself, chat, eavesdrop. Learning a few names and faces can put things on a much friendlier basis.

If your throat is dry, take a warm drink. Ironically, speakers are usually given a pitcher of ice water. A cold drink will contract throat muscles, but a warm one will relax them.

The Delivery

Take a deep breath. Concentrate on the audience, not on yourself. Make eye contact. Smile, Even if there are 300 people in the room, speak to one person at a time.

Engage your audience as much as possible. Draw them in and get them to nod in agreement with what you are saying.

Although you should never memorize your whole speech, there are two parts you should memorize: your opening line and your closing line. Knowing exactly how you will launch your speech will reduce anxiety. Knowing how you can bring your speech to an effective close lets you be more relaxed and responsive during your speech.

Be sensitive to your audience. Do not ignore their needs by hurrying through your speech. Watch them. If they seem confused, bored, overheated, or agitated, stop. Find out where the problem lies. You may need to open a window, close a door, take an unscheduled stretch break, give them an individual exercise, or allow them to make comments and ask questions.

If you are giving a presentation to your classmates and you have only one picture, chart, or model, do not pass it around the group while you are talking. It is too distracting. Either make a copy for everyone, convert the material into a slide, or offer to make it available after the session for anyone who wants a closer look.

Audio-visual aids make a presentation more interesting and enhance learning. Pictures are literally worth a thousand words. The audience will forget 90 percent of your words but will remember pictures and the thoughts behind them.

Handouts can supplement information and reduce the need for note taking. If you are only going to discuss three aspects of cerebral palsy, you may want to make a list of "Twenty Facts About Cerebral Palsy" with a suggested reading list. Participants like something in their hands that they can take home.

If someone asks a question and you don't know the answer, say, "I don't know the answer, but I will have it for you tomorrow." If you make a mistake, admit it. If someone challenges your information, be ready to cite sources. If he or she persists, offer to meet later to compare and contrast information. If someone is argumentative, don't become defensive. Say, "That is a very interesting point of view. I would like to continue this discussion when there is more time."

WORDS DELIVERED ON PAPER

When you have to deliver words on paper, you can follow many of the same principles that apply to delivering words in person. First, *know your audience*. Who is going to read this paper? Write for the reader.

Decide on the purpose of the paper. Are you attempting to inform, persuade, or entertain?

Consider the importance of the assignment. Is this a daily exercise, or a paper that will constitute half of your grade? The amount of time you invest should be proportional to the amount of benefit you expect to receive.

Next, choose a topic. Choosing is not as difficult as narrowing that topic down to a manageable size. Before you begin writing "Communicable Diseases Through the Ages" (a topic that would fill 10 volumes), talk to your instructor. You will probably end up writing something more like "Measles from 1910 to 1920." If you follow your instructor's advice and suggestions, success is almost guaranteed because your instructor is your reader.

Once you and your instructor have agreed on the topic, draft a brief outline. Then head for the library and the librarian. Librarians will direct you not only to current guides for nursing literature, but also to computer services that can generate a list of all relevant articles published in the last few years. The fee is nominal and well worth it if your time is short.

Usually your problem will be identifying *quality* articles. Occasionally the problem is finding an adequate *quantity* of articles. A couple of years ago I attended a meeting of the American Association for the Advancement of Science. One of the sessions, *"The Oldest Old,"* was to focus on people over the age of 85 (the fastest-growing segment of the population). When the sociologists who did the presentation went to the library to do research, they literally found nothing there. The subject was *too recent.*

Provided what you need is in print, your librarian can help you find it. Even if your school is small and your library is limited, the librarian can arrange interlibrary loans. Books and journals can be sent from major health science libraries.

Before you spend much time reading any article, scan it. Titles are often misleading, and many that appear relevant are not.

As you read, watch for recurring themes, major issues, milestones, facts, and figures. Take notes on index cards. Keep track of questions that need answering.

Before you begin writing, refine your outline. Reorganize it and make it as comprehensive as possible. Decide which information carries the most weight. Prioritize objectives just as you did when preparing your speech. What is the most important idea or piece of information? The second most important? The third?

Floor It

Let your fingers fly when you write the first draft. Pay no attention to spelling, punctuation, phrasing, or logic. Scribble thoughts as fast as they occur to you. Whether you write or type, leave wide margins and plenty of space between lines where you can rewrite or add information.

Set the paper aside. Sleep on it. The next morning, work it over. Edit, reorganize, expand. Strive for simple words and short sentences.

Write a second draft. If possible, let 2 or 3 days elapse, then work it over again. Reading your paper aloud is often helpful.

Sometimes when you work long and hard on a project, you cannot see its fatal flaws. Let a friend check your paper for readability, logic, and content. Ask for a double check on spelling and punctuation. If you use a word processing program with a spell checker, be sure to use it.

Formats for footnotes and bibliographies are varied. What is in vogue at one school will be inappropriate at another. Ask your instructor for guidelines. In an emergency, just follow the format in one of your recommended textbooks. As long as you are consistent in the way you handle references, you will not lose more than a couple of points.

When you print the final draft, use good-quality white paper (at least 20-pound, preferably with rag content). Make sure each page has a number and your name. Do a professional-quality job on the title page and the cover. Neatness does count.

Finally, the only thing better than delivering your paper on time is delivering it ahead of schedule.

No matter what route you take after nursing school, skills as a speaker and writer will always help you.

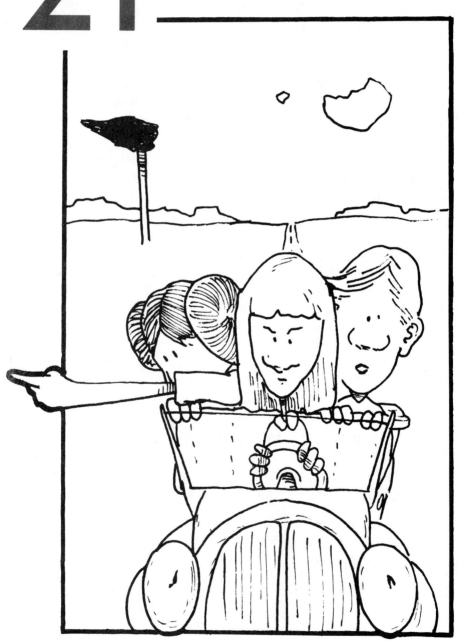

IN THE DRIVER'S SEAT

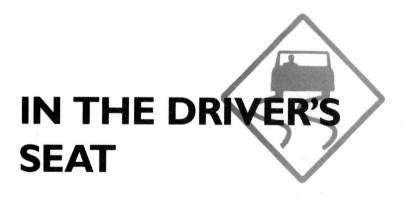

"Experience is the name everyone gives
to his mistakes."
            —Oscar Wilde

A few feet off the interstate, the exit split into north-bound and southbound lanes. The driver ahead of me was obviously unsure which lane was the "right" lane. Before he could make up his mind, he impaled his car on the lane divider.

If he had it to do over again, I am sure he would agree that even the "wrong" decision would have been better than no decision. He may have had to drive a little out of his way, but he would have arrived in one piece.

In a moving vehicle, decision time is limited. To be a good driver, you need a ready mind and a steady hand. You need to size up situations quickly, make decisions, and take action.

The same is true of nursing.

When you are in the driver's seat, you take full responsibility for your actions. When you make an error, you must take the consequences. Even if some backseat driver gave you a bum steer, the citation will be issued to you.

The same is true of nursing.

Professionally speaking, when you are in the driver's seat, you take full responsibility for your actions. When you make an error, and you will, do not waste time making excuses. Face up to your responsibility. Learn from the experience. Then drive on.

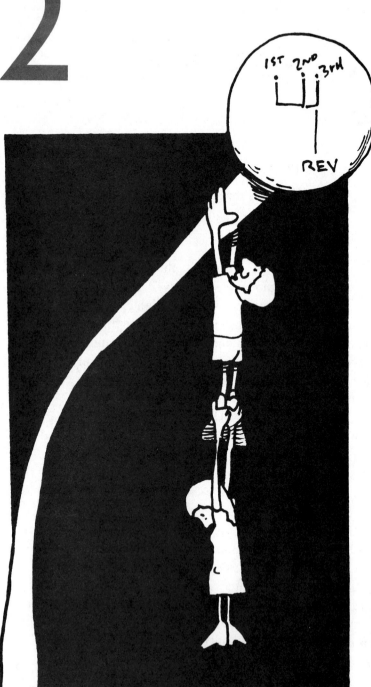

SHIFTING GEARS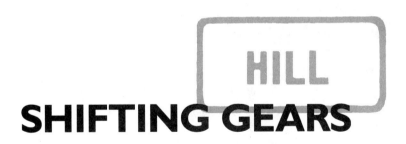

"I feel as I always have, except for an
occasional heart attack."
                    —Robert Benchley

Going back to school after several years absence can be a
real jolt to the system. The song goes, "I will never pass this
way again," and yet here you are back in school at 25, 30, 40,
or 50 years of age.

Consider what happened to my sister. She is a business
whiz. When a golden opportunity appeared, she did not see
the need to finish college. She signed on with a rapidly expanding company and, through a combination of sheer talent
and incredibly hard work, rose to a vice president's position.
She was on the fast track and confident she had it made.
Until . . . her company merged. She found herself out on the
street with several other top-level managers.

She quickly discovered it was impossible to get a comparable position without proper academic credentials. Oh there
were jobs available but not the career opportunities she
wanted. For example, one representative told her his company would not even interview her for a *secretarial* position
without a bachelor's degree. She soon found herself back in
school—a little older, a little wiser.

People who find themselves back in school at midlife are
called "mature" students. Whether this is a first career venture, a move to enhance career options, or a complete career
change makes little difference. In addition to the academic
challenge, there are a multitude of other stressors.

VINTAGE VEHICLES

Mature students don't worry about a date for homecoming. They worry about coming home and finding the babysitter has quit. The cupboard is bare, the toilet is overflowing, the dog is in heat, and the mortgage is due. Meeting obligations means continually making tough choices and uncomfortable compromises.

Many mature students have to commute. They can't relocate their families so they "dislocate" themselves.

"I was a full-time student at the university with a husband 200 miles away who claimed he couldn't cook for himself. I drove 200 miles on Friday to cook, clean, be the ideal wife on Saturday and Sunday. I drove back Sunday evening and spent the whole night studying for the week. Both grades and marriage came out intact, but I was physically and mentally exhausted."

A long drive to and from school can be a grueling experience. Here is how one student came to enjoy her roadwork.

"I spend 12 hours away from home at least 5 days a week. My 'spare time' is spend driving 2 hours each day to and from school. At first I resented the drive. Now I love it. I can sing all four parts to the choir songs. I love to listen to the news and the games. I recognize certain cars and trucks; we honk and wave. I share a common bond with their drivers. Life has so many perks if you just look for them. My 2 hours behind the wheel have become a gift instead of a burden."

Maintaining a positive attitude and accepting the drive as part of the price of higher education will shorten the road. Don't waste time and energy resenting reality. Go with it.

The road to nursing always goes uphill. If you want to make it to the top, you have to shift to a lower gear and lighten your load as much as possible. This is especially true of married students and/or those with children regardless of their age.

Married men have an advantage. They have wives. Married women have a disadvantage. They *are* wives.

Being a wife-mother-student means going into overdrive. After spending all day in class and clinical, you race home (driven by guilt), toss in a load of laundry, start dinner, vacuum the living room, balance the checkbook, check the kids' homework, walk the dog, and listen to an instant replay of your husband's day at work. When you finally get everyone bedded down for the night, you tiptoe to the kitchen table, spread out your books, and study until past midnight. The next morning you wake up tired and already behind schedule.

Many women fail to make the grade in nursing school because they refuse to lighten their load. They vow that nothing will change. They try valiantly to do everything just as before, but they fall farther and farther behind. Women drive themselves too hard.

They've Found Something that Can Do the Work of Ten Men ...

Participants at a Midwestern nursing management conference included approximately 100 women and *only one man*. All held demanding jobs in middle and upper management. The afternoon session dealt with the Superwoman complex— the compulsion to do everything perfectly, from cooking to cleaning to parenting to advancing a career.

The man, who was still a bachelor, was amazed at what he heard. He didn't see how the women could manage to do everything at work and everything at home. It had never occurred to him that he should do his own housework. As soon as he was employed, he had hired someone to come in twice a week.

It doesn't occur to men to do their own housework. It doesn't occur to women *not* to do their own housework. Time to shift!

After that conference, many of those nurse-managers probably hired housekeeping help. As a student you may not be able to afford help, yet you cannot afford to be without it. If you can't hire it, you have to commandeer it.

Just as it never occurred to the male manager to do his own housework, it will probably never occur to your husband to do *his* own housework. Studies show that husbands of working wives do no more household chores than husbands of nonworking wives. Chances are that this holds true for children too. If you want your family's help around the house, you will have to be the one who says so.

Make lists of essential household chores and let family members choose which ones they prefer to do. Divide the ones nobody wants and assign them on a rotating basis. Have some chores available for extra credit. These pay bonuses over allowances.

Dancing in the Dust

An Iowa student found she could get the whole family to pitch in for 1 hour every Saturday morning. They turned on rock-and-roll music, and all six of them danced through the house doing their assigned chores.

If dancing housecleaners don't measure up to your exacting standards, relax your standards. In fact, if you are going to survive nursing school, you have to relax, period.

Family members can feel threatened as your friends, interests, lifestyle, and priorities shift. There may be some anger, fear, jealousy, and resentment. There can also be new joy, pride, fun, and adventure.

Who *Is* This Person?

Nursing absorbs so much time and attention that one man complained he had to make an appointment just to see his wife. A lot of the romance and spontaneity seemed to have gone out of their relationship. Their solution? They stopped thinking of their times together as "appointments" and began thinking of them as "dates." It revitalized their marriage.

The spouse always plays a critical role in the student's success or failure.

"As a diploma nurse the push is to get a degree and move on to a master's. When I was married with three children and a full-time job, I started back to school. My husband was very nonsupportive. 'That is more time away from me and the children.' I felt guilty about that too, but I was also angry. I had supported my husband through his last year of college and 4 years of postgraduate work. I went ahead with school but eventually dropped out. I guess the guilt and nonsupport weakened me. I'm now divorced with a full-time job, three children, less money, and going to school because my job requires a bachelor's."

How supportive is your spouse?

NO SUPPORT   FULL SUPPORT

☐ __ __ __ __ __ __ __ __ __ ☐

Be honest. Support is not just talk, it's ACTION! As a student prepared to head for the library one evening, her husband groaned, "Do I have to babysit again?" She snapped back, "No, you don't have to babysit. The only children here tonight will be yours!"

When long-established patterns are disrupted, when standard operating procedures are violated, tensions mount and tempers flair. In many ways the whole family goes back to school. Everyone is learning, adjusting, and adapting.

As you return to school, it's nice to have the support of friends and family. Not every student is that fortunate.

"Upon deciding I wanted a career—not just a job—I pledged to give it my all. My parents and relatives did not understand. My husband has ALWAYS been supportive, but comments from those 'outside' our lives really hurt. They would say things like 'You sure are neglecting your husband' or 'It's too bad you can't spend more time together' or 'YOU can do that; YOU don't have children.' I decided to set my own goals and do what was needed to attain them. I have been successful. Whether other people support me or not, I made the decision that this is MY life and I'm doing these things for ME!!!"

How important is it for you to have the approval of family and friends? Can you stand alone? Can you say with this student, ". . . it is MY life and I'm doing these things for ME!!!" If you can, your chances of success are much greater.

Kiddie Car

The more support you have from your children, the better your chances of surviving nursing school. Let them know that things will be different—not necessarily better or worse, just different. Help your family make the shift.

Involve your children as soon as possible and as much as possible. Talk to them about your school. Take them to the library, to your classroom, to the nursing skills laboratory, and to the hospital. Children are much more comfortable when they can visualize where their parents are.

Make your children NURSE KITS. Toss in syringes, tongue blades, bandages, finger cots—whatever you can scrounge. Buy them a stethoscope of their own.

One family had "study hall" around the dining room table from 7:00 to 8:30 P.M. Another family had each member go to a separate room and close the door for a "quiet hour."

To survive you will need a private place where you can study. Privacy is something mothers are not supposed to need. Moms are supposed to be accessible 24 hours a day, 7 days a week, 365 days a year. Shift!

Go to your room. Close your door for 1 hour. Let an older child or your spouse handle problems and answer questions. When you emerge from study time, be ready to give your full, undivided attention to the family. If they know you will be really available at a certain time, they will permit you a study hour.

Even though you can't do everything together, you can do the important things together. What are the most important things? Ask your child. "What's one thing you would like us to do together today?" It may be having a special story read, hosting a tea party in the tree house, shopping for new tennis shoes, going to the zoo, working on a school project, or playing Monopoly. Let your children help plan special evenings, weekend outings, or vacation events.

Recognize that although you can do *anything*, you cannot do *everything*. You have to make concrete decisions.

For example, while driving across the country one summer, we decided to take a 200-mile detour and spend 1 day in a city where we had lived for several years. How could we see everyone in just 24 hours? We couldn't. So each of us chose the one person we most wanted to see. When we entered the city limits, we phoned the four people and made arrangements to see them. Then we drove to our old neighborhood and fit in other people and activities as we could. We left bright and early the next morning feeling very satisfied and happy that we had made the detour.

WOMEN DRIVERS

One of the most popular workshops I teach is designed for women who are trying to do it all, have it all, and be it all. I call it "Walk-On-Water Women" (WOW for short). I ask participants to describe a situation in which two or more of their roles are in conflict. Many of the examples involve women who are back in school trying to be good wives, good mothers, good daughters, good neighbors, good employees, and good students SIMULTANEOUSLY! It is exhausting.

In her fascinating book called *Sequencing*, Arlene Rossen Cardozo talks about women who have chosen to do it all but not simultaneously. These women have had the foresight or the fortitude or the good fortune to have completed their education, established themselves firmly in careers, and then chosen to experience full-time mothering. I would call this sequencing with a capital "S." And I personally know of only one woman who has managed to pull this off.

For the rest of us—the frantic, the frazzled—who are trying to do it all simultaneously, I would like to recommend sequencing with a small "s." It begins with acknowledging that you cannot be in two places at once.

"Sometimes I feel torn—I'm working and in school, and on weekends I need to clean house, do laundry, scrub floors, cut grass, etc., etc., etc. My husband wants to do something fun for the weekend. I feel the need to spend time with him and the family, but then I have twice as much work to do when I return home—tired kids, dirty laundry, messy house. Most of the time I give in and then pay the price later for the fun. But again, sometimes I don't enjoy myself much because I know what's waiting for me when I get home— AND return to work and school THE NEXT DAY! Sometimes I resent my husband for not being able to see the work that needs to be done at home."

Here is another student with the same conflict but a much healthier way of handling it:

"When do I feel stressed? When behind in classes and housework and needing to do a million things at home! Like last Saturday when Hubby and kids wanted to go to the cottage for a day but I didn't—

I wanted to get caught up. This caused a conflict between my needs and theirs. After a 'discussion' the family went without me. I got everything done and felt good about the day. They came home having had a great day, and we wondered why we had argued."

In nursing school your social life will be sharply curtailed. With little time for family, you will have almost no time for friends. Say goodbye to dinner parties and hello to potlucks. You can also invite friends over just for dessert or have a taco party to which everyone brings their favorite ingredient. True friends don't come for the food; they come for the fun of being together. And true friends won't mind if your house was cleaned by six rock-and-roll dancers.

Socialize with your classmates and their families. Families can compare notes, swap stories, sympathize with each other, and help solve problems.

Always have contingency plans. If the babysitter falls through, who is the backup person? If one of the children is sick, who will stay home? If the car breaks down, what alternate transportation is available? Contingency plans include a spare house key hidden in the flower pot, a spare lasagna in the freezer, a spare $20 bill under the mattress, and a spare uniform in the closet. Then you can shift at a moment's notice.

MAN BEHIND THE WHEEL

Being a man in a traditionally female career calls for double clutching. Some men fail to make the grade because they look at nursing with the idea that if a woman can do it, *any* man can do it. They think they can conduct business as usual and learn nursing in their spare time. In no time they find themselves with four flats and no spare.

Some men falter because they can't shift into a student role. They cannot surrender their independence. Some can't shift into scientific thinking. Others can't shift into a nurturing mode. A few cannot cope with being surrounded, supervised, and instructed by women.

It is tough to be in the minority. Instead of thinking only 3 percent of nurses are men, tell yourself there are well over 50,000 men in nursing. And you're going to be one of them!

BLACK AND WHITE

Black students, especially those enrolled in predominantly white colleges or impersonal, large research universities, appear to be at high risk. (Susan H. Jones: "Improving Retention and Graduation Rates for Black Students in Nursing Education: A Developmental Model," *Nursing Outlook*, Vol. 40, No. 2, March/April 1992, pp. 78–84.)

Those most likely to drop out are often the first in their family to attend college. Their high school experience was "marginal," and they doubt their ability to actually attain a degree. Under enormous academic, financial, and social pressure, they report feeling ignored, alienated, and alone.

If you find yourself caught in this pressure cooker, where can you find support? Chi Eta Phi, the black nursing sorority, alumni groups, and local chapters of the National Black Nurses' Association.

PROFESSIONAL DRIVERS

Whether male or female, black or white, young or old, you have to be able to shift gears when you enter the hospital. You must switch to your professional gear. For instance, people two or three times your age will be asking *you* for advice. They will tell you things they wouldn't tell their best friend, their spouse, or their cleric. You must respect these confidences, always protecting your patients' privacy and dignity.

With some practice, shifting from the personal to the professional mode becomes almost automatic. There are times, however, when that shift must be a conscious, deliberate decision.

For example, one nurse had some nagging personal problems that began interfering with her ability to concentrate at work. One day she noticed a large laundry basket parked outside the operating room area. As she passed by, she decided to dump her personal problems mentally into that basket. At the end of her shift she mentally picked up her personal problems. Turning her personal life off during working hours made her happier and more productive. After work, even though she "picked up" her problems again, she felt better able to carry them. She approached her personal life with a new freshness and was able to resolve her problems in a short time.

MAKING THE GRADE

Mature students are often more uptight about grades than their younger counterparts. They feel driven to excel. Perhaps it is one way to justify all the time, energy, and money being diverted into school. Perhaps they want to set a good example for their own children. Whatever their motivation, they don't want to be good students, they want to be great.

Grades can become more important than learning. I know it's true. I've been there. I have spent a major portion of my life as a student. I feel like the fellow who quipped, "I've been in school so long I know things that just ain't so."

Like other overachievers, I have my own private grading system. If I get an A, I'm not always sure I earned it. I know I could have done more, learned more. If I get a B, I'm upset because Suzie-Q got an A, and I know I'm just as smart and worked just as hard as she did. If I get a C, I'm destroyed. For a highly competitive person like me, that's an automatic failure.

When I approached graduate school, I wanted things to be different. First of all, I wanted to combine psychiatric and pediatric nursing, but no such program existed. I devised one of my own. I took electives, did extra reading, and arranged my clinical assignments to reflect my private agenda. While conforming on the surface, below the surface I was busily doing my own thing.

I knew if I let grades influence me, I would neglect my own priorities. So I chose not to know my grades. To receive your grades at the University of Washington, you had to turn in a set of stamped, self-addressed envelopes. I didn't turn in any envelopes. I did not see my grades the entire time I was in graduate school. I figured if I were in academic trouble, someone would tap me on the shoulder and tell me to shape up. If

I were doing OK, then it was just that—OK! I wouldn't get sidetracked by the pursuit of perfection.

During my fourth quarter I discovered what a liberating experience it had been. Evidently one faculty member was a notoriously unfair grader. My fellow students were up in arms, ready to get tar and feathers. I just smiled to myself. I didn't know my grade. It honestly didn't matter to me. I had learned what I wanted to learn and had already moved on to other things.

Sometimes the only way to get where YOU really want to go is to shift gears and "brake" with old habits and traditions. Do whatever it takes to make sure learning is more important than grading.

BUYING AMERICAN OR JAPANESE?

When educational psychologists gave an unsolvable math problem to groups of Japanese and American children, they uncovered one key as to why our academic achievement is so much lower. The American kids struggled briefly and then gave up. The Japanese kids kept working, apparently believing that if you persist you can solve any problem.

Hard work is the key to success. Yet many Americans believe the key to success is inborn talent. Either you have it or you don't. So say educational psychologists Jim Stigler and Harold Stevenson, coauthors of *The Learning Gap* (New York, Simon & Shuster, 1992). They say our obsession with natural talent and innate ability has produced kids who give up easily. In fact, many Americans believe people who work hard in school must lack ability.

If you believe people are born smart, chances are you're a quitter. If you believe people are made smart, you'll knuckle down, persevere—and succeed! You'll know what Thomas Edison knew, that genius is 1 percent inspiration and 99 percent perspiration.

Being able to shift gears quickly is essential if you are to survive nursing school. From now on, you will have to shift more; "shiftless" students won't make it.

23

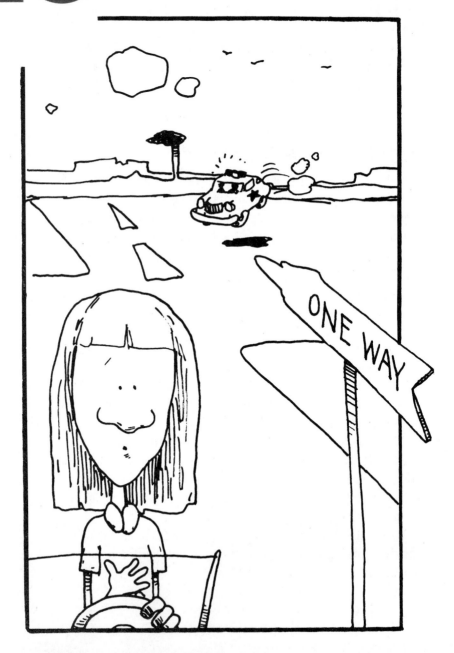

MOVING 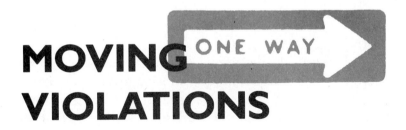 VIOLATIONS

"Well, Mrs. Upjohn, I guess I know my business. Of course, that's just a guess on my part."

—Groucho Marx,
A Day at the Races

The summer before I went to nursing school, I worked a couple of months as a nurses' aid. I received no training or orientation. I was dumped directly on a busy floor during the evening shift. The nurse in charge would teach me the ropes as she had time.

I ran errands, fetched water, delivered dinner trays, and then was assigned to help patients get ready for bed, which included giving backrubs. The charge nurse told me to use lotion and powder.

My first "victim" was Maxine, a patient quite debilitated with multiple sclerosis. I smeared lotion all over her broad back and then liberally sprinkled powder on top. The two ingredients combined to form a lumpy paste. The more I rubbed, the worse it got.

Maxine shrieked, "Good grief, girl, what do you think you're doing!?" I replied, "Making pie crust." She burst into laughter.

I explained it was my first night, and I really had no idea of what I was doing. Immediately she became my teacher. I learned a lot of basics from Maxine, including how tough it is to be a patient. She wrote to me while I was a nursing student, and whenever I got home, I went to see her. She died shortly after I was graduated.

Fortunately, you won't be tossed into the hospital in such a casual way. Before you hit the road, you will receive a lot of instruction.

Most of us had a driver's education course, and before we were allowed on the road, we spent hours reading, studying, and testing. There were films, demonstrations, discussions, and simulators to approximate driving conditions so that we could rehearse responses to all sorts of situations. When we passed the first part of the course, we were allowed to get behind the wheel of a specially equipped car. At our side sat an instructor using a dual-control system to keep us from making any costly errors. After we passed both written and driving exams, our licenses were granted. For the first time we were allowed to drive solo.

Nursing education follows much the same pattern. Before you are allowed to touch a patient, you spend hours reading, studying, testing, and rehearsing all sorts of technical procedures. If you are successful in the nursing skills laboratory, an instructor will accompany you to the patient for a real test of your ability. The instructor is there to protect you and your patient from any costly error. If you pass the patient test, you are allowed to do the procedure solo.

Being able to pass the "patient test" is crucial. If you fail the clinical portion of the course, you fail the course. There is no grade averaging here. Even straight-A students who fail clinical are out. The course must be repeated.

Mastering the skills and procedures of nursing practice is essential. To survive in nursing you must be able to use your hands as well as your head.

Of the students who botch their clinical component, only one in a thousand is a complete klutz. The others are usually ill-prepared or suffer acute anxiety attacks that interfere with their performance.

To be well-prepared you need to make the most of your time in the nursing skills lab. While waiting for your turn, you can learn a lot from your classmates. Keep alert. Watch every movement. Listen to the instructor's comments and the responses of your classmates. Envision yourself in your classmate's place. Feel the equipment in your hand. Anticipate each step. Recite the rationale to yourself. Concentrate.

USING YOUR HEAD

Sports experiments have repeatedly confirmed the value of "synthetic" experience. For example, in a classic study students were divided into three groups and then tested on their ability to shoot free throws. For almost 3 weeks after the initial testing, group 1 practiced shooting free throws, group 2 did nothing related to basketball, and group 3 spent 20 minutes every day *imagining* they were shooting free throws. At the final test group 2 showed no improvement, but groups 1 and 3 improved 24 percent and 23 percent, respectively. Studies like this indicate that the human nervous system cannot distinguish between an actual experience and a vividly imagined one.

Picture Perfect

If you picture yourself failing, you double your chances of failure. If you picture yourself succeeding, you double your chances of success. So picture yourself doing the procedure and doing it perfectly, with precision and finesse. Mentally rehearse.

To control your anxiety, take slow, deep breaths. Focus on the patient and his or her needs. Recognize that sweaty palms, cold feet, butterflies in the stomach, and lightheadedness are normal symptoms of anxiety. Once the procedure is complete, they will disappear.

Be assured that you will never be permitted to practice a procedure on a patient that you haven't perfected in the skills lab. Remember, the instructor will be right by your side to coach you and to keep you from doing harm.

The first time you perform any procedure is nerve-racking at best. Some students keep trying to postpone the inevitable. They keep their heads down and stand at the back of the group, hoping they won't be chosen. Although it is possible to get through nursing school with minimum experience, it is not possible to get through with *no* experience.

Every time you postpone doing a procedure, anxiety builds until it reaches panic proportions. Confidence is the only cure, and confidence comes from competence. Competence comes from experience, and experience often comes the hard way. So keep your head up, stand at the front of the group, and volunteer.

I asked nurses what they would suggest students do to help take the terror out of clinical experience. Here is what they said:

> "Remember that you are a student and there to learn. So ask questions and don't be afraid of not being perfect."

> "Take a deep breath and say, I'm OK! I can do it!"

> "Believe in yourself. Don't sweat the small stuff!!!"

> "Don't ever be afraid to ask how to do something or admit you don't know an answer. We've all been in your shoes."

> "We were all students once—remind us of what it's like. Ask for help and guidance."

> "Don't tell the patient this is your first time. It isn't. You've practiced this over and over in the classroom."

> "Just put yourself in the patient's place and think about how you would like to be treated."

> "Relax. Be calm. The patient is a person just like you."

> "Determine what will REALISTICALLY happen if you goof or screw up. The patient won't die and neither will you."

> "Blow the situation so out of proportion that you'll laugh. Picture yourself and the patient as cartoon characters."

> "Remember every nurse from the director of nursing on down had to take this first step."

"Don't let your instructor intimidate you. Remember, she was once a terrified student like you."

"Actually, your instructor wants you to pass/excel even more than you do. Think about it! If you don't look good, she doesn't look good. She's cheering for you."

"Pray."

"The first time is always terrifying. Go on—do it! The second time it feels better and works better."

"Realize anyone can make a mistake. There is no such thing as a bad experience. Always look for the positive. What have I learned from this?"

"Don't be afraid or embarrassed to try. Even if you blunder, remember doing is learning. It leads to confidence. Grab every experience you can!"

To get adequate experience, you may not only need to volunteer, you may have to fight to volunteer. Time in the clinical area is limited, and the procedures available are at a premium. You may get only *one* opportunity to perform a certain procedure. Once is not enough to build confidence or competence. To get more than minimum experience, make sure the staff knows which procedures you need to practice and which ones you are allowed to do solo. Make sure they know you are ready, willing, and able.

In driving and in nursing the most serious infractions are moving violations. To keep from being labeled "Unsafe At Any Speed," practice, practice, practice.

24

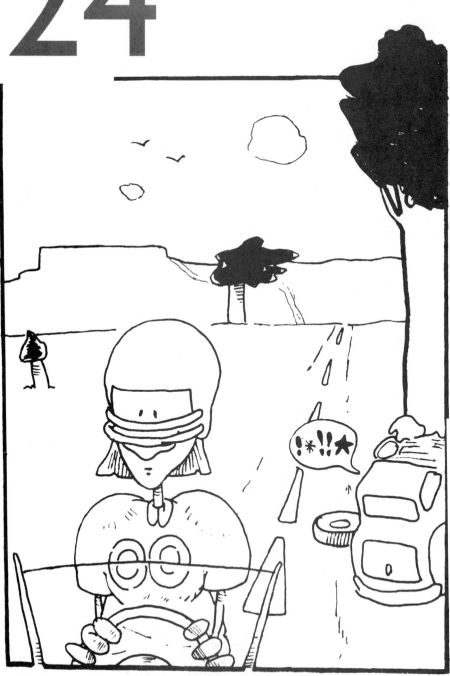

DEFENSIVE DRIVING

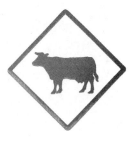

"There are no liberals behind steering
wheels."
> —Russell Baker,
> *Poor Russell's Almanac*

When you drive defensively, you protect yourself by watching out for the other guy. In many ways watching out for the other guy is the very essence of nursing. Caring for and about others is our business. We have traditionally been more concerned about the rights of others than about our own rights.

During the 1970s, delineating "the other guy's" rights became a national pastime. Every conceivable group emerged from that decade with a "bill or rights." Patients had several champions. For example, see the pages following for the American Hospital Association's version of a patient's bill of rights.

A PATIENT'S BILL OF RIGHTS

1. The patient has the right to considerate and respectful care.

2. The patient has the right to and is encouraged to obtain from physicians and other direct caregivers relevant, current, and understandable information concerning diagnosis, treatment, and prognosis.

Except in emergencies when the patient lacks decision-making capacity and the need for treatment is urgent, the patient is entitled to the opportunity to discuss and request information related to the specific procedures and/or treatments, the risks involved, the possible length of recuperation, and the medically reasonable alternatives and their accompanying risks and benefits.

Patients have the right to know the identity of physicians, nurses, and others involved in their care, as well as when those involved are students, residents, or other trainees. The patient also has the right to know the immediate and long-term financial implications of treatment choices, insofar as they are known.

3. The patient has the right to make decisions about the plan of care prior to and during the course of treatment and to refuse a recommended treatment or plan of care to the extent permitted by law and hospital policy and to be informed of the medical consequences of this action. In case of such refusal, the patient is entitled to other appropriate care and services that the hospital provides or transfer to another hospital. The hospital should notify patients of any policy that might affect patient choice within the institution.

4. The patient has the right to have an advance directive (such as a living will, health care proxy, or durable power of attorney for health care) concerning treatment or designating a surrogate decision maker with the expectation that the hospital will honor the intent of that directive to the extent permitted by law and hospital policy.

Health care institutions must advise patients of their rights under state law and hospital policy to make informed medical choices, ask if the patient has an advance directive, and include that information in patient records. The patient has the right to timely information about hospital policy that may limit its ability to implement a legally valid advance directive.

5. The patient has the right to every consideration of privacy. Case discussion, consultation, examination, and treatment should be conducted so as to protect each patient's privacy.

6. The patient has the right to expect that all communications and records pertaining to his/her care will be treated as confidential by the hospital, except in cases such as suspected abuse and public health hazards when reporting is permitted or required by law. The patient has the right to expect that the hospital will emphasize the confidentiality of this information when it releases it to any other parties entitled to review information in these records.

7. The patient has the right to review the records pertaining to his/her medical care and to have the information explained or interpreted as necessary, except when restricted by law.

8. The patient has the right to expect that, within its capacity and policies, a hospital will make reasonable response to the request of a patient for appropriate and medically indicated care and services. The hospital must provide evaluation, service, and/or referral as indicated by the urgency of the case. When medically appropriate and legally permissible, or when a patient has so requested, a patient may be transferred to another facility. The institution to which the patient is to be transferred must first have accepted the patient for transfer. The patient must also have the benefit of complete information and explanation concerning the need for, risks, benefits, and alternatives to such a transfer.

9. The patient has the right to ask and be informed of the existence of business relationships among the hospital, educational institutions, other health care providers, or payers that may influence the patient's treatment and care.

10. The patient has the right to consent to or decline to participate in proposed research studies or human experimentation affecting care and treatment or re-

quiring direct patient involvement, and to have those studies fully explained prior to consent. A patient who declines to participate in research or experimentation is entitled to the most effective care that the hospital can otherwise provide.

11. The patient has the right to expect reasonable continuity of care when appropriate and to be informed by physicians and other caregivers of available and realistic patient care options when hospital care is no longer appropriate.

12. The patient has the right to be informed of hospital policies and practices that relate to patient care, treatment, and responsibilities. The patient has the right to be informed of available resources for resolving disputes, grievances, and conflicts, such as ethics committees, patient representatives, or other mechanisms available in the institution. The patient has the right to be informed of the hospital's charges for services and available payment methods.

These rights can be exercised on the patient's behalf by a designated surrogate or proxy decision maker if the patient lacks decision-making capacity, is legally incompetent, or is a minor.

In addition to general rights for general patients, all sorts of highly specialized subgroups had their own lists of rights: the disabled, the retarded, the pregnant, the dying, ad infinitum.

As lists of rights proliferated and legislation was passed, nursing turned its attention to drafting lists of responsibilities. The American Nurses' Association drafted a code of ethics, and the National League for Nursing developed "Nursing's Role in Patient Rights."

ANA CODE FOR NURSES

1. The nurse provides services with respect for human dignity and the uniqueness of the client, unre-

stricted by considerations of social or economic status, personal attributes, or the nature of health problems.

2. The nurse safeguards the client's right to privacy by judiciously protecting information of a confidential nature.

3. The nurse acts to safeguard the client and the public when health care and safety are affected by the incompetent, unethical, or illegal practice of any person.

4. The nurse assumes responsibility and accountability for individual nursing judgments and actions.

5. The nurse maintains competence in nursing.

6. The nurse exercises informed judgment and uses individual competence and qualifications as criteria in seeking consultation, accepting responsibilities, and delegating nursing activities to others.

7. The nurse participates in activities that contribute to the ongoing development of the profession's body of knowledge.

8. The nurse participates in the profession's efforts to implement and improve standards of nursing.

9. The nurse participates in the profession's efforts to establish and maintain conditions of employment conducive to high quality nursing care.

10. The nurse participates in the profession's effort to protect the public from misinformation and misrepresentation and to maintain the integrity of nursing.

11. The nurse collaborates with members of the health professions and other citizens in promoting community and national efforts to meet the health needs of the public.

From American Nurses Association, © 1985. Reprinted with permission.

NURSING'S ROLE IN PATIENT RIGHTS

1. People have the right to health care that is accessible and that meets professional standards regardless of the setting.

2. Patients have the right to courteous and individualized health care that is equitable, humane, and given without discrimination as to race, color, creed, sex, national origin, source of payment, or ethical or political beliefs.

3. Patients have the right to information about their diagnosis, prognosis, and treatment—including alternatives to care and risks involved—in terms they and their families can readily understand, so that they can give their informed consent.

4. Patients have the legal right to informed participation in all decisions concerning their health care.

5. Patients have the right to information about the qualifications, names, and titles of personnel responsible for providing health care.

6. Patients have the right to refuse observation by those not directly involved in their care.

7. Patients have the right to privacy during interview, examination, and treatment.

8. Patients have the right to privacy in communicating and visiting with persons of their choice.

9. Patients have the right to refuse treatments, medications, or participation in research and experimentation, without punitive action being taken against them.

10. Patients have the right to coordination and continuity of health care.

11. Patients have the right to appropriate instruction or education from health care personnel so that they can achieve an optimal level of wellness and an understanding of their basic health needs.

12. Patients have the right to confidentiality of all records (except as otherwise provided for by law or third-party payer contracts) and all communications, written or oral, between patients and health care providers.

13. Patients have the right of access to all health records pertaining to them, the right to challenge and to have their records corrected for accuracy, and the right to transfer all such records in the case of continuing care.

14. Patients have the right to information of the charges for services, including the right to challenge these.

15. Above all, patients have the right to be fully informed as to all their rights in all health care settings.

From National League for Nursing, Nursing's Role in Patient Rights, New York (Pub. No. 11–1671), 1977.

Nursing wanted to do more than conform to the letter of the law—we wanted to conform to the spirit of the law. We took our responsibility for the rights of others very seriously. We still do.

In fact, nurses are so involved in protecting the rights of others that we often forget we have rights of our own. Perhaps that is why my list of "Ten Basic Rights for Women in the Health Professions" attracts so much attention.

1. You have the right to be treated with respect.
2. You have the right to a reasonable workload.
3. You have the right to an equitable wage.
4. You have the right to determine your own priorities.
5. You have the right to ask for what you want.
6. You have the right to refuse without making excuses or feeling guilty.
7. You have the right to make mistakes and be responsible for them.
8. You have the right to give and receive information as a professional.
9. You have the right to act in the best interest of the patient.
10. You have the right to be human.

It is not the rights themselves, but the very idea that nurses *have* rights, that is novel.

As a nursing student you may be surprised to find that you have rights, too. For example, you have the right to see your educational records and to challenge information that you believe is inaccurate. Your records are to be kept private. With the exception of the registrar and your current instructor, no one should have access to your files without your permission. These rights are not at the discretion of the school but are legislated by Congress (Buckley Amendment). As expressed by the NSNA,

"Every member of a nursing school must be held accountable for his/her action, be it an instructor, administrator or a student. NSNA believes that every school of nursing should have a written agreement between its students, faculty and administration."

This may be a good time to check into student rights on your campus. Rights are usually tucked away among the written rules, regulations, and requirements. They should include protection from capricious grading, incompetent instructors, and unsafe environments, as well as providing specific guidelines for grievance procedures. To drive defensively you should know your rights long before you have to use them.

Even when rights are carefully spelled out, however, we know that there is a big difference between conforming to the letter of the law and conforming to the spirit of the law. Take the example of "informed consent." This is a paper that patients are asked to sign before surgery or treatment is undertaken. The document was developed to protect patients' rights. The intent was to make sure physicians instructed patients about their diagnoses, alternate treatments available, and potential risks or complications as well as potential benefits.

THE STUDENT BILL OF RIGHTS AND RESPONSIBILITIES

The following Student Bill of Rights and Responsibilities was adopted by the NSNA House of Delegates in April 1975.

1. Students should be encouraged to develop the capacity for critical judgment and engage in a sustained and independent search for truth.

2. The freedom to teach and the freedom to learn are inseparable facets of academic freedom: students should exercise their freedom with responsibility.

3. Each institution has a duty to develop policies and procedures which provide and safeguard the students' freedom to learn.

4. Under no circumstances should a student be barred from admission to a particular institution on the basis of race, creed, sex, or marital status.

5. Students should be free to take reasoned exception to the data or views offered in any course of study and to reserve judgment about matters of opinion, but they are responsible for learning the content of any course of study for which they are enrolled.

6. Students should have protection through orderly procedures against prejudiced or capricious academic evaluation, but they are responsible for maintaining standards of academic performance established for each course in which they are enrolled.

7. Information about student views, beliefs, and political associations which instructors acquire in the course of their work should be considered confidential and not released without the knowledge or consent of the student.

8. The student should have the right to have a responsible voice in the determination of his/her curriculum.

9. Institutions should have a carefully considered policy as to the information which should be a part of a student's permanent educational record and as to the conditions of this disclosure.

10. Students and student organizations should be free to examine and discuss all questions of interest to them, and to express opinions publicly and privately.

11. Students should be allowed to invite and to hear any person of their own choosing, thereby taking the responsibility of furthering their education.

12. The student body should have clearly defined means to participate in the formulation and application of institutional policy affecting academic and student affairs.

13. The institution has an obligation to clarify those standards of behavior which it considers essential to its educational mission and its community life.

14. Disciplinary proceedings should be instituted only for violations of standards of conduct formulated with significant student participation and published in advance through such means as a student handbook or a generally available body of institutional regulations. It is the responsibility of the student to know these regulations. Grievance procedures should be available for every student.

15. As citizens and members of an academic community, students are subject to the obligations which accrue them by virtue of this membership and should enjoy the same freedoms of citizenship.

16. Students have the right to belong or refuse to belong to any organization of their choice.

17. Students have the right to personal privacy in their living space to the extent that the welfare of others is respected.

18. Adequate safety precautions should be provided by schools of nursing, for example, to and from student dorms, adequate street lighting, locks, etc.

19. Dress code, if present in school, should be established by student government in conjunction with the school director and faculty, so the highest professional standards possible are maintained, but also taking into consideration points of comfort and practicality for the student.

20. Grading systems should be carefully reviewed periodically with students and faculty for clarification and better student-faculty understanding.

From National Student Nurses' Association, Inc.: The Bill of Rights and Responsibilities for Students of Nursing, New York, 1978, NSNA.

If you read consent forms from your local health care institutions, you will quickly see that they are written in terms only physicians and lawyers can understand. You will not be surprised to learn that (a) many patients think they *have* to sign, and (b) the vast majority think the purpose is to protect physicians' rights, not their own.

By obtaining the patient's signature, the physician has "consent." He has conformed to the letter of the law. If the patient is truly "informed," then the doctor has conformed to the *spirit* of the law as well.

Most of us want to live up to the spirit of the law. All of us *have* to live up to the letter of the law if we want to maintain licensure and avoid litigation.

Until recently, nurses were seldom named as defendants in lawsuits. There were two reasons for this. First, nurses' salaries were so low that it literally did not pay to sue us. Second, nurses were assumed to be merely carrying out orders. We were not held accountable.

Today we find nurses named in lawsuits right along with doctors and hospitals because salaries have risen substantially and because nurses now carry malpractice insurance. We are profitable targets. In addition, nurses are no longer seen as robots who mechanically carry out doctors' orders. The law perceives us as fully functioning professionals and holds us responsible for our actions and for our failure to act. In fact, the law requires nurses to exercise more judgment than some physicians, administrators, or nurses may deem acceptable.

The legal implications of nursing care are so complex that whole books are devoted to the subject. Professional journals frequently run articles dealing with legal issues in nursing, and many have regular columns on the subject. Law has become a popular graduate school option for nurses, and the number of nurse-attorneys is growing rapidly.

To avoid the courtroom you must take a road that is paved with paperwork: charting, care plans, anecdotal notes, incident reports, discharge summaries. Although paperwork is time-consuming, it should never be treated as trivial.

Donna Lee Guarriello, a nurse-attorney, provided a graphic illustration of the importance of paperwork. The case involved a young woman who suffered a cerebral hemorrhage and became permanently paralyzed after the birth of her first child. Initially Guarriello intended to name the nurse together with two physicians in the lawsuit. After all, the nurse had spent 8 hours caring for the patient. During that time the patient's condition had steadily deteriorated. Apparently the nurse had been negligent.

After reading the nurse's notes, however, the attorney decided not to sue her. According to the chart, the nurse had repeatedly tried to get proper attention and treatment for the patient. She had phoned the attending physician suggesting he transfer the patient to intensive care. He refused. She contacted her supervisor. When the attending physician did not come to the hospital and did not return her subsequent phone calls, she arranged for another obstetrician and a resident to see the patient. Unfortunately, they refused to countermand the orders of the attending physician.

Everything was thoroughly, objectively, and professionally documented in the patient's chart. The nurse had not been negligent—quite the contrary. Paperwork did not help the patient, but it did save the nurse.

Always remember: defensive driving begins and ends with paperwork. Pay close attention to your instructor when it comes to documenting patient care. Don't waste time complaining about the amount of paperwork involved in nursing. Learn to do it efficiently and effectively. Your professional life may depend on it.

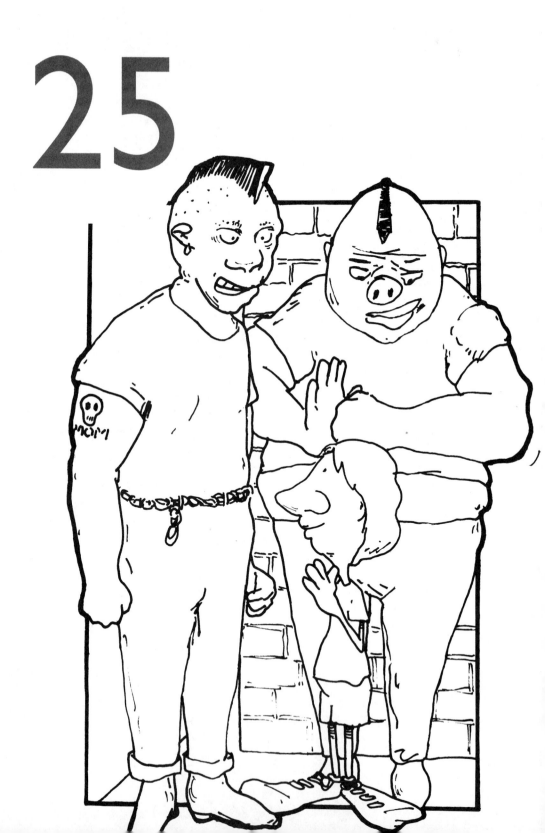

25

STREET SMART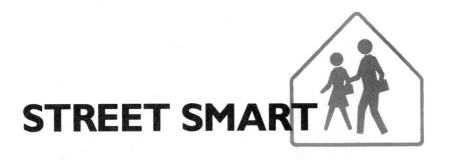

> "Start each day with a smile and get it
> over with."
> —W.C. Fields

You are traveling through a tough neighborhood. People here are sick and angry. And that's just the faculty! You have the staff and patients to deal with, too. What a shame everyone seems to gang up on students. You would swear no one remembered what it was like to be the new kid on the block.

Don't they remember what it was like to be a student? Yes, they do. They remember exactly what it was like. Most went through hell and high water to become nurses. Many are still convinced it is the only way to initiate you into the profession. Before you can be a member, you have to prove your mettle. You have to show that you can stand up and take it like a nurse.

The only way to become part of any gang is to pay your dues. In nursing that means working together shoulder to shoulder, 40 hours a week, 50 weeks a year, for years and years. So when you enter the clinical setting, don't be surprised to feel like an outsider. You *are* an outsider. You are not part of the gang. If you are lucky, the staff will treat you like a guest. If you are unlucky, they will treat you like a trespasser.

Your instructor may or may not be part of the gang. Some faculty members have joint appointments, meaning they are employed by both the educational and the health-care institutions. They have real-life responsibilities for both the clinical unit and the classroom.

Most instructors, however, have a sole employer: the school. Consequently, their status on the clinical unit may be almost equivalent to that of a student. Some instructors are warmly welcomed; others are barely tolerated. Given enough time and effort, faculty can earn a place in the gang. If your instructor has done so, count yourself fortunate.

Nursing service and nursing education are often at odds. Each has a different mission, and sometimes they appear at cross purposes. Education strives for the ideal, whereas service must struggle with what is real.

For all practical purposes you and your instructor are just passing through. The staff lives here. This is *their* turf, hard-fought and hard-won on a daily basis.

If you want to survive in this neighborhood, do not criticize the staff. Over the years you will learn that there is a big difference between book smart and being street smart.

To pave the way for the best possible clinical experience, you not only need to *give* a good first impression, you also need to *get* a good first impression.

GETTING A GOOD FIRST IMPRESSION

Unfortunately, every hospital is different, and every unit in every hospital is different. Just when you begin to feel comfortable in one clinical setting, they make you rotate to another. Each new rotation begins with orientation—a rapid tour accompanied by a continuous stream of rules, regulations, policies, and preferences.

By the end of the tour some students are so anxious that they can no longer tell a crash cart from a laundry cart. Their senses are jammed by the sights, sounds, and smells of the unit. Instead of reducing their anxiety, orientation seems to accentuate it.

If orientation gives you a headache instead of a head start, you may want to make a preorientation visit to the facility and to the unit on which you are assigned. Many students recommend visiting your new clinical setting a few days early. To get a general feeling of the place, they suggest you sit in the lobby, spend time in the patient waiting areas, eat in the cafeteria, and just ride the elevators. Make a mental map of the way to your unit, the nursing office, the major departments, laboratories, and clinics. Students recommend visiting your specific unit on evenings because they are usually less hectic than the day shift. Whatever time of day you choose, you are cautioned to avoid change-of-shift periods.

GIVING A GOOD FIRST IMPRESSION

Make sure you arrive on the clinical unit clean, pressed, and appropriately dressed. Wear your name tag and look like you mean business. The more professional you look, the more professional courtesy will be extended to you.

Stand tall and walk confidently. Look people in the eye. Smile. Be energetic but not hyperactive. Control nervous gestures like cracking your knuckles or twisting your hair.

Introduce yourself and ask for the person in charge. Give your name, rank, and serial number. State your purpose and ask permission to come on the unit.

"I'm Sherry Jackson, a second-year student, and I'll be on this unit beginning Monday. Would it be OK if I looked around a little? I'd like to get my bearings before orientation."

If you want to get along with the gang, always show respect for their territory and their time. Remember the staff nurses' names. Call them by the title they prefer. Be friendly. Be sincere.

Let the staff do most of the talking. Be a good listener. Encourage them to talk about themselves and their professional experiences. You can learn a lot vicariously.

Ask their advice. Respect their opinions. Avoid arguing, criticizing, or complaining.

Get them to reminisce about their student days. They have some wonderful tales to tell. Listening to their war stories will reassure you about the future. If they survived, so can you. Recalling their past may also make them more sensitive to your present needs.

Always be ready to do a little more than required. Volunteer to give a hand without being asked. Say please and thank you. Common courtesy is all too uncommon.

PATIENTS PLEASE

Often first impressions are formed even before you meet your patient. If you spend too much time studying the chart before going to his room, you may picture him as a series of problems, not as a person. If a staff member says, "So you're the one who got stuck with Mr. Elmers," you will have a much different first impression than if you are told, "Mr. Elmers is a terrific fellow. You are going to enjoy caring for him." Try to suspend judgment. Realize that first impressions or second-hand impressions may be more harmful than helpful.

The approaches that you used to make a good first impression on the staff can also help you make a good first impression on the patient—for example, dressing appropriately, looking professional, and controlling nervous gestures.

Before entering the patient's room, knock. Ask permission to enter. Respect what precious little turf the patient has.

Focus on the patient instead of on his tubes, dressings, or machinery. Look him in the eye. Pull up a chair and sit down. Introduce yourself and ask what name he prefers to be called. Tell him who you are and when you will be caring for him.

Before leaving ask if he has any questions or if there is anything you can do for him. A simple act like making sure the call bell is within reach, fetching fresh water, dialing the phone, fluffing the pillows, or finding out when he is scheduled for surgery can win him over.

HEARING WITH YOUR EYES

Street-smart students know that body language often contradicts verbal language. A patient winces yet says, "I'm fine." The head nurse says, "Welcome to 4 West," but her arms are folded tightly across her chest and her body is rigid.

Learning to listen with your eyes as well as your ears helps you interpret what is happening more accurately. By studying nonverbal communication, you will learn how to read people.

For example, did you know that leaning your head on one hand indicates interest, but leaning on both hands indicates boredom? Did you know that crossed arms are a sign of a closed mind, that locked ankles indicate worry or uncertainty, that a hand covering the mouth shows a lack of confidence and a reluctance to talk? Did you know that when people lie they tend to have rapid eye movements, lick their lips, rub their eyes, or scratch nervously?

As you learn more about body language, you will understand why it is not so much what you say but how you say it that counts. You observe one doctor who calls, "How are you?" from the doorway and another who goes to the bedside, touches the patient's shoulder, and asks the same question. The words are identical but the effect is totally different. Which doctor really cares about the answer? Which doctor is going to get the more accurate response?

When trying to make a good impression, you choose your words carefully. Make the same careful choices when it comes to appearance, posture, and gestures. Actions do speak louder than words. Just ask any street-smart student.

26

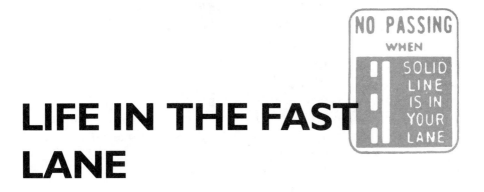

LIFE IN THE FAST LANE

"Now, *here*, you see, it takes all the running
you can do, to keep in the same place. If
you want to get somewhere else, you
must run at least twice as fast as that!"
—Lewis Carroll,
Through the Looking Glass

Well, it's time for one last lap around the track. And the last lap may be the hardest. *"People told me each year got easier—not true! Each year is harder."*

If you are approaching your final year, you may appreciate these tips from students who were only days away from graduation. To prepare for that last go-round, they suggest you:

"Spend the summer reviewing *everything* you've covered."

"Get all nonessentials (anything that doesn't pertain to school) out of the way before entering that last year."

"Get a summer job in a hospital. That experience will help you make the most of your last year."

"Try to identify your niche in nursing and request clinical experience in that area."

At the beginning of your final year, most students say, "really kick it into high gear" and "give it all you've got!"

"Try to get every possible experience. Keep in mind how quickly a year goes. Get everything you can NOW!"

"Challenge *yourself*. Don't worry about grades."

"Keep your eye on your goal. Make every moment count."

"Quit your job. Don't work if at all possible. Focus all your energies on learning anything and everything."

"Read every nursing journal you can get your hands on."

"Join all the professional organizations and clubs you can."

"Attend in-service programs at the hospital whenever possible."

"Get involved. Become politically, financially, and professionally informed—do not have tunnel vision about your profession."

"Work hard . . . it will all be over soon."

Other students suggest you ease up a bit on the accelerator:

"Relax! This is what you've been waiting for. You're about to accomplish a very important goal."

"Enjoy your last year. When it's over, you're going to miss it."

"Relax. You know more than you think you do."

"Take time out to reflect on all you've accomplished."

No matter how tough things get, don't quit! A student from Texas said, "If I can make it, you can make it!" She's right. Every year about 80,000 nursing students "make it." You might as well be one of them. So . . .

"Don't give up! Keep fighting!"

"Hang on!"

"Think POSITIVE!"

"Keep swimming, Babe, the shore is in sight!"

The good news is that you are about to graduate. That's also the bad news. If you graduate, you have to face state board examinations. The mere mention of state boards—the final to end all finals—produces something akin to mass hysteria. These near-graduates suggest that you not become obsessed by state boards but rather prepare for them confidently and systematically.

"First things first. Concentrate on school."

"Write for information on state board testing dates."

"Buy a review book and pledge to spend 15 minutes a day with it."

"Form a group specifically to study for boards."

"Don't panic. Your instructors will help you. After all, if you don't look good, they don't look good."

"Enroll in a review course. They are available." (A list of Mosby's review books and courses appears in Appendix A.)

As graduation approaches and attentions shift to finding a job, seniors advise you to:

"Start surveying employment opportunities early. Read the nursing career guides as well as the classified ads in newspapers."

"Form a job-search club. Critique each other's resumés. Discuss local and national career opportunities."

"Talk with recruiters and write to as many hospitals as possible for information. Xerox anything you get, and share it with classmates. You're all in this together."

"Look for a mentor. See if there's an opportunity to work alongside a nurse you admire."

"Look for a hospital that offers an extensive, comprehensive internship program for new grads."

"Talk to last year's graduates and find out how they like their jobs. Ask them for suggestions. Is there anything they wish they had done differently in their senior year?"

"Remember, nursing is loaded with possibilities. Keep an open mind about specialization, new directions, and professional goals. You may be surprised!"

27

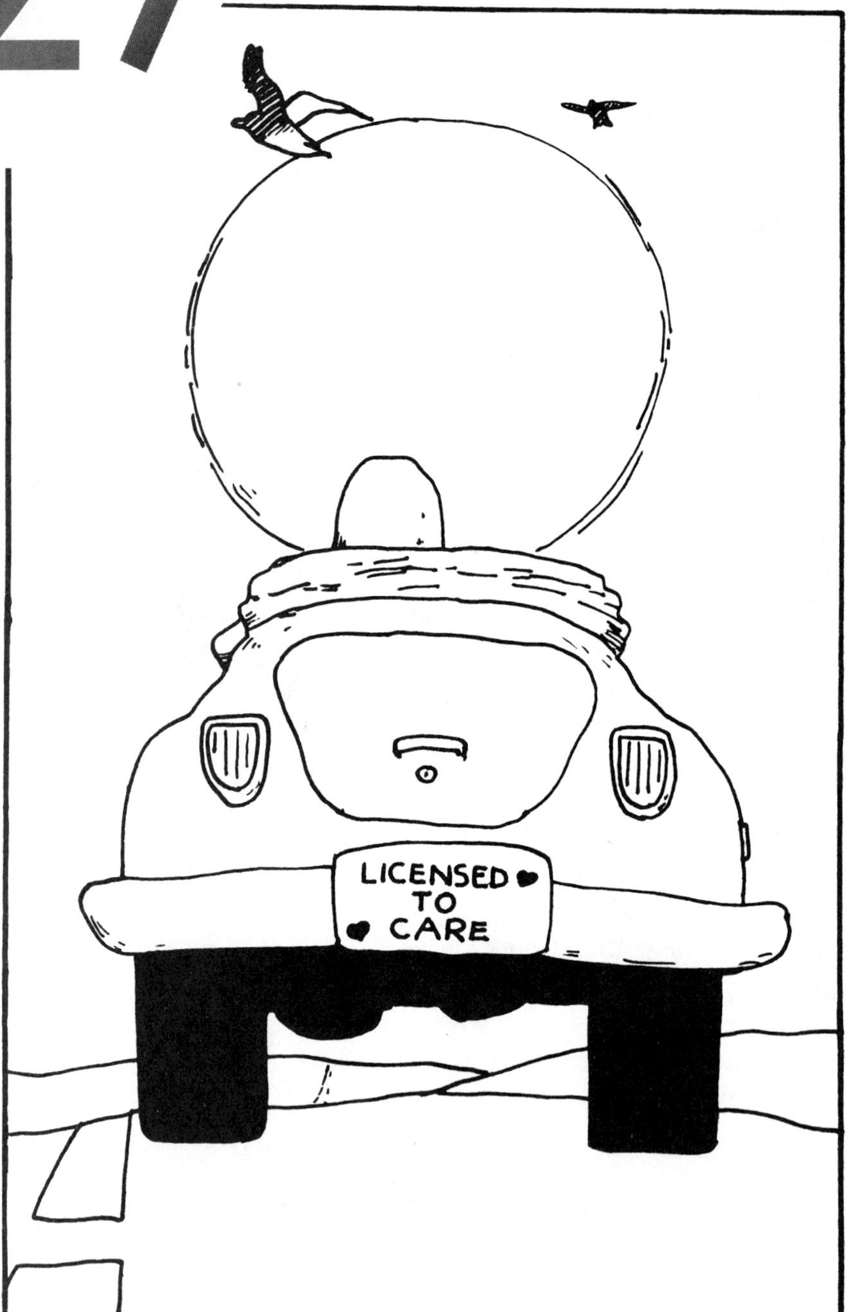

ARE WE THERE YET?

"O Captain! my Captain! our fearful trip is done!
The ship has weather'd every wrack,
the prize we sought is won,
The port is near, the bells I hear,
The people all exulting."

—Walt Whitman,
O Captain! My Captain!

Once you have graduated and passed the state board exams, you have arrived. And yet . . . the journey is just beginning.

You surrender your learner's permit and pick up a professional license. One moment you are a thoroughly experienced student. The next moment you are a thoroughly *in*experienced professional.

But, if you have gotten this far, YOU CAN DO ANYTHING.

APPENDIXES

A   RESOURCES FOR NCLEX REVIEW

B   GRIEVANCE PROCEDURE GUIDELINES

C   COMMON PREFIXES AND SUFFIXES USED IN
    NURSING

D   SOURCES OF SCHOLARSHIPS AND LOANS

E   QUESTIONS AND ANSWERS ON THE
    COMPUTERIZED NCLEX-RN EXAM

F   U.S. STATE AND TERRITORIAL BOARDS OF NURSING

G   U.S. AND CANADIAN NURSING ORGANIZATIONS

H   SPECIALIZED NURSING ORGANIZATIONS IN THE
    UNITED STATES AND CANADA

Resources for NCLEX Review available from Mosby

AJN/Mosby Nursing Boards Review,
9th edition, 1994

This is designed as a review tool and study guide for students preparing to take the NCLEX-RN in the U.S. or the Comprehensive Licensure Examination in Canada. Essential content from all core clinical areas is presented in outline format with a nursing process focus. Sample tests include 374 questions presented in the stand-alone format used on the Boards.
Price: $27.95
Book code: 07781

The AJN/Mosby Question and Answer Book,
4th edition, 1994

This resource presents nearly 2000 questions to provide practice for the NCLEX-RN and Canadian Comprehensive Licensure Examination. Questions are organized by core clinical areas and grouped by health problems. Two sample exams are included. Answers include rationales to reinforce learning and clarify misconceptions.
Price: $22.95
Book code: 07780

Mosby's Comprehensive Review of Nursing,
14th edition, 1994 (15th edition to
publish October 1995)

Dolores F. Saxton, Patricia M. Nugent, and Phyllis K. Pelikan

This review book and study guide is designed to prepare students for the NCLEX-RN examination in the United States and the Comprehensive Licensure Examination in

Canada. It features content review outlines and questions for all clinical areas. The five-step nursing process is integrated into the content reviews. Two 375-question examinations are included for additional practice. Also included is a computer disk which contains an additional 100 practice questions with rationales.

Price: $28.95
Book code: 24847

Mosby's AssessTest: A Practice Exam for RN Licensure, unsecured version

Dolores F. Saxton, Phyllis K. Pelikan, Patricia M. Nugent, and Selma R. Needleman

Mosby's AssessTest is a practice test that features 375 questions constructed according to the NCLEX-RN test plan. It evaluates performance based on nursing process, client needs, cognitive level, and clinical area. Each student receives a list of questions answered incorrectly as well as a booklet containing question classifications, correct answers, and rationales for all answer choices. The *AssessTest* is updated annually.

1995 version (available October 1994):
Price: $26.95
Book code: 24779
1996 version (available October 1995):
Price: $26.95
Book code: 24837

Mosby's Review for NCLEX-RN, second edition, 1995

Dolores F. Saxton, Phyllis K. Pelikan, Patricia M. Nugent, and Selma R. Needleman

This review book provides over 2,200 questions to help students prepare for the NCLEX-RN exam. Questions for each core clinical area (medical-surgical, maternity, pediatric, and psychiatric-mental health nursing) are grouped by subsection (pharmacology, body systems, and nutrition). Two comprehensive examinations with rationales for all answer choices are also included. Along with the text is a computer

disk containing 100 additional questions to provide practice answering questions on the computer.
Price: $22.95
Book code: 24777

Mosby's NCLEX Review

Dolores F. Saxton, Phyllis K. Pelikan, and Judith Green

This IBM-compatible computer disk contains 400 new practice questions with rationales for all answer choices. It can be used in either test or tutorial mode. Feedback is provided for the overall score as well as subscores for clinical area, nursing process, and client needs.
Price: $29.95
Book code: 24915

Pass NCLEX-RN! videotape and booklet, 1994

This video/booklet package includes three sections to help you prepare for the computerized NCLEX exam: (1) an overview of the test plan; (2) five case scenarios, each accompanied by a series of sample questions to illustrate the content and format of questions included on the exam; and (3) test-taking tips and strategies.
Price: $9.95
Book code: 24831

Pass NCLEX Review course

This 4-day, multi-media review course covers the medical-surgical, obstetric, pediatric, and psychiatric components of the NCLEX exam, as well as test-taking strategies and stress reduction techniques designed to improve test performance. Practice questions assist in sharpening test-taking skills.

The course is offered in December/January and May/June. For specific dates and locations of courses, call 1–800–826–1877.

Grievance Procedure Guidelines

NSNA believes that the basis of "rights" and "procedures" is a contractual agreement between the school and student that clearly spells out the expectations and responsibility of students, faculty, and administration, and that any agreement must include a procedure for dealing with infringements of the contract.

The following guidelines were developed by the NSNA Board of Directors in January 1975.

1. Before a set of grievance procedures can be discussed, a Student Bill of Rights and Responsibilities must be devised. It is suggested that students use the guidelines developed by NSNA for this. The Bill should be a written statement mutually agreed upon by both faculty and students.
   Rationale: The Student Bill of Rights and Responsibilities is the guideline on which the grievance committee can depend to help in making a decision on the issue at hand.

2. The procedure for handling grievances should be a well-defined, written statement. Both faculty and students should have equal representation in the development of such a procedure.
   Rationale: It is necessary to have a procedure that both students and faculty will support.

3. Once grievance procedures are developed, students should be made aware of the existence of these procedures at orientation.
   Rationale: Students should know what steps they can take if a situation should come up where their rights are infringed upon.

4. The grievance committee should be composed of an equal representation of students and faculty, with a minimum ratio of four to four.

Rationale: Equal representation with at least eight on the committee provides for broader range, more objective opinions.

   a. Student members on the committee should be composed of at least one representative from each class. These members should be elected by the student body.

Rationale: Students from different classes often have differing outlooks and viewpoints on a situation. Election insures that student members have the support of and are representative of the student body.

   b. Faculty members on the committee should be chosen by the faculty, except in the situation as described in #12.

Rationale: The faculty should choose representatives.

5. There should be a written statement, drawn up by student and faculty representatives, which indicates the amount of power the grievance committee has, and the types of situations that fall under the committee's jurisdiction.

Rationale: Defining this will help to support the decisions made by the committee.

Some suggestions:

   a. Enforcement of the Student Bill of Rights and Responsibilities.

   b. Review student evaluations of courses and faculty, and make recommendations to the appropriate people. Same principle here as in #10.

   c. Review curriculum and grading system, and initiate change as necessary.

   d. Review dress code (if any).

   e. Review other grievances, not necessarily in Student Bill of Rights.

6. The committee should meet regularly—at least once a month, and all students should be informed as to the date, time, and place of these meetings.

Rationale: To give students an opportunity to air grievances that are not of an emergency nature.

7. Accurate records, including complete minutes, and in individual cases, a verbatim record, shall be kept on file for all meetings of the committee. These minutes should be signed by at least one faculty member and one student on the committee.

   Rationale: To serve as evidence of the committee's action should there ever be any question about it. Also to serve as a precedent for future committee action should a similar case ever arise.

8. Any student shall have the right to ask for an "emergency meeting" of the grievance committee on matters that are crucial and cannot wait until the regularly scheduled meeting.

   Rationale: To provide a means of handling grievances in a "crisis" situation.

9. State and local constituents of the National Student Nurses' Association should make their board members available for advice and support for any student initiating a grievance, and this available support should be publicized.

   Rationale: Students filing complaints need positive reinforcement in their efforts. Also nursing students need to know that their Student Nurses' Association is truly interested in and representing them and their concerns.

10. As a preliminary step, the student's case will be heard by a subcommittee of the regular grievance committee. This subcommittee will consist of two faculty members and two students. If the subcommittee cannot satisfactorily solve the grievance, they will report to the main grievance committee which will then hear the case and take action as necessary.

    Rationale: Often grievance cases can be adequately handled by persons who are impartial. This would conserve the workload of the entire committee. Also, this subcommittee can help the committee have greater insight and understanding of the cases that are presented to them.

11. The student appearing before the grievance committee should have the right to have a representative or advisor of his/her choice with him/her at the meeting.

    Rationale: To allow the student to have the necessary resources he/she needs in order to adequately present his/her case. Also, sometimes students who are emotionally involved with a case are not able to present it in the way they would like.

12. If the grievance is against a member of the committee, the student should have a right to ask the member to abstain from participation in the committee while his/her grievance is being considered. The committee should then appoint someone to take that member's place.

    Rationale: To protect the student from a biased decision by the committee, and allow the student more freedom to express his/her opinion.

13. A mediator should be allowed to sit on the committee. This should be someone who is neither a faculty member nor a student, but is closely associated with nursing. The mediator should be without vote and refrain from expression his/her opinion. The purpose of the mediator is to make sure that each member on the committee has an equal opportunity to speak and that full and fair review of the facts takes place.

    Rationale: To prevent an individual or group on the committee from becoming too powerful and domineering.

14. Reasonable evidence and background material concerning the case should be submitted to the committee at least three days prior to the date when the case is to be discussed.

    Rationale: To allow the committee adequate time to examine the facts prior to being required to make a decision on the matter.

15. Any charges against the student or faculty member should be in writing and be made available to both the committee and the student at least three days before his/her scheduled appearance.

    Rationale: To give the student adequate time to prepare a defense against charges.

16. The student should be given full opportunity to present evidence and witnesses that are relevant to the issue at hand. He/she should also be given the opportunity to question any witnesses against him/her and also be informed of any evidence against him/her and its source.
Rationale: To make sure that the facts are being presented fully and fairly.

17. The student should be allowed to continue class as usual until the committee has reached a decision.
Rationale: To avoid the possibility of falling behind in school while the case is being considered, and avoid any delaying tactics that may be employed to prevent the student from returning to class.

18. Group grievances should be presented to the committee by one representative of that group. That representative may then appoint a consultant to appear with him.
Rationale: To provide an organized, systematic way of dealing with group grievances.

19. The decision of the committee should be made in writing to the student within two weeks of hearing the case.
Rationale: To assure a fair review and conclusion of the student's case.

20. Decisions made by the committee are final, that is, immediately enforced by both faculty and students, except in cases with legal implications (e.g., discrimination, in which the student plans to take the case to court).
Rationale: To avoid delay in enforcing the decision.

21. Provisions should be made for a "right of appeal," in which the student can take *his* case to the Dean or a governing board of the school. However, until the "appeals board" reaches a decision, the student is still bound by the "grievance committee's" decision.
Rationale: To allow the student a solution to take if he feels that his case has been unfairly handled by the committee.

From National Student Nurses' Association, Inc.: The Bill of Rights and Responsibilities for Students of Nursing, New York, 1978, NSNA.

Common Prefixes and Suffixes Used in Nursing

PREFIXES	MEANING
a-, an-	without, not
ab-	away from
ad-	to, toward
adeno-	gland
aero-	air
ambi-	around
amphi-	about, on both sides, both
ampho-	both
ana-	up, back, again, excessive
angio-	vessel
ano-	anus
ante-	before, forward
anti-	against, counteracting
ap-, apo-	from, separation
arterio-	artery
arthro-	joint
bi-	double
bili-	bile
bio-	life
bis-	two
brachio-	arm
brady-	slow
broncho-	bronchus
cardio-	heart
cata-	down, under, lower, against
cepha-, cephalo-	head
cerebro-	cerebrum
cervico-	neck
chole-	gall, bile
cholecysto-	gall bladder
chondro-	cartilage
circum-	around
co-	together

PREFIXES	MEANING
com-, con-	with, together
contra-	opposite, against
costo-	ribs
cranio-	head
cyto-	cell
cysto-	bladder
de-	away from
demi-	half
derm-, derma-	skin
dia-	between, through, apart, across, completely
dis-	from
dorso-	back
dys	difficult, abnormal
e-, ex-, exo	out, away from
ec-	out from
ecto-	on outer side, situated on
electro-	related to electricity
em-, en-	in
encephal-	brain
endo-	within
entero-	intestines
epi-	upon, on
equi-	equal
eryth-	red
extra-	in addition to, outside of
ferro-	iron
fibro-	fiber
fore-	in front of, before
gastro-	stomach
glosso-	tongue
glyco-	sugar
hemi-	half
hemo-, hema-	blood
hepa-, hepato-	liver
histo-	tissue
homo-	same
hydro-	water
hyper-	high, excessive
hypo-	low, decreased
hyster-, hystero-	uterus

PREFIXES	MEANING
im-, in-	in, into, not
infra-	below
inter-	between
intra-	within
intro-	in, into, within
juxta-	near, close
laparo-	abdomen
laryngo-	larynx
latero-	side
leuk-	white
lympho-	lymph
macro-	large
mal-	poor, bad
mast, masto-	breast
medio-	middle
mega-	large, great
meno-	menses
meta-	beyond, after, change
micro-	small
mono-	single
multi-	many
myelo-	spinal cord, bone marrow
myo-	muscle
naso-	nose
neo-	new
nephro-	kidney
neuro-	nerve
nitro-	nitrogen
noct-	night
non-	not
ob-	in front of, against
oculo-	eye
odonto-	tooth
oophoro-	ovary
ophthalmo-	eye
opistho-	behind, backward
orchio-, orchido-	testes
ortho-	straight, normal
os-	mouth, bone
osteo-	bone
oto-	ear

PREFIXES	MEANING
ovario-	ovary
pan-	all
para-	beside, along with
path-	disease
ped-	child, foot
per-	by, through
peri-	around
pharyngo-	pharynx
phlebo-	vein
photo-	light
pneumo-	air, lungs
pod-	foot
poly-	many, much
post-	after, behind
pre-, pro-	before, in front of
proct-, procto-	rectum
pseudo-	false
psych-	mind
pyo-	pus
pyro-	fever
quadri-	four
radio-	radiation
re-	back, again
reno-	kidney
retro-	backward
rhino-	nose
sacro-	sacrum
sclero-	hard, hardening
semi-	half
spleno-	spleen
steno-	narrowing, construction
sterno-	sternum
sub-	under
syper, supra-	above, excess
sym-, syn-	together
tachy-	fast
teno-	tendon
thyro-	thyroid
trache-	trachea
trans-	throughout, across
tri-	three
ultra-	beyond

PREFIXES

PREFIXES	MEANING
un-	not, reversal
uni-	one
uretero-	ureter
urethro-	urethra
uro-	urine
vaso-	blood vessel
veno-	vein

SUFFIXES

SUFFIXES	MEANING
-able	able to
-algia	pain
-cele	swelling, tumor
-centesis	surgical puncture
-cide	destructive, killing
-cule	little
-cyte	cell
-ectasia	expansion, dilation
-ectomy	excision
-emia	blood
-esis	action
-form	shaped like
-genesis	origin, formation
-graph	writing
-iasis, -ism	condition
-itis	inflammation
-ize	to treat
-lith	stone
-lysis	disintegration, dissolution
-malacia	softening
-megaly	enlargement
-meter	measuring instrument
-oid	resemblance, likeness
-oma	tumor
-opathy, -pathy	any disease of
-orrhaphy	surgical repair
-osis	disease
-ostomy, -stomy	to form an opening
-otomy, -tomy	incision into
-penia	deficiency, decrease
-phage	ingesting
-phobia	fear

Sources of Scholarships and Loans

First, check the financial aid office at your school. For undergraduate financial aid, here are the addresses of state programs:

Alabama
205-269-2700
Student Assistance
  Program
Alabama Commission
  on Higher
  Education
One Court Square,
Suite 221
Montgomery, AL
  36197

Alaska
907-465-2962
Alaska Commission on
  Postsecondary
  Education
Box FP, 400
  Willoughby
Juneau, AK 99811

Arizona
602-255-3109
Commission for
  Postsecondary
  Education
3300 North Central
  Avenue, #1407
Phoenix, AZ 85012

Arkansas
501-371-1441
Department of Higher
  Education
1220 West Third
  Street
Little Rock, AR 72201

California
916-445-0880
Student Aid
  Commission
PO Box 942845
Sacramento, CA 94245

Colorado
303-866-2723
Colorado Commission
  on Higher
  Education
1300 Broadway,
  Second Floor
Denver, CO 80203

Connecticut
203-566-2618
Department of Higher
  Education
61 Woodland Street
Hartford, CT 06105

Delaware
302-571-3240
Delaware
  Postsecondary
  Education
  Committee
State Office Building
820 North French
  Street
Wilmington, DE 19801

District of Columbia
202-727-3685
DC Office of
  Postsecondary
  Education Research
  and Assistance
1331 H Street NW,
  #600
Washington, DC 20005

Florida
904-488-4095
Office of Student
  Financial
  Assistance
Department of
  Education
Florida Education
  Center
Tallahassee, FL 32399

Georgia
404-493-5444
Georgia Student
  Finance Authority
2082 East Exchange
  Place, #200
Tucker, GA 30084

Hawaii
808-948-8213
Hawaii State
  Postsecondary
  Education
  Commission
Bachman Hall, Room
  209
244 Dole Street
Honolulu, HI 96822

Idaho
208-334-2270
State Board of
  Education
650 West State Street
Boise, ID 83720

Illinois
321-948-8550
708-948-8550
State Scholarship
  Commission
Client Support
  Services
106 Wilmot Road
Deerfield, IL 60015

Indiana
317-232-2350
State Student
   Assistance
   Commission
964 North
   Pennsylvania Street
Indianapolis, IN 46204

Iowa
515-281-3501
Iowa College Aid
   Commission
201 Jewett Building
Ninth and Grand
Des Moines, IA 50309

Kansas
913-296-3517
Board of Regents,
   State of Kansas
Suite 609, Capitol
   Tower
400 West Eighth
   Street
Topeka, KS 66603

Kentucky
502-564-7990
Higher Education
   Assistance
   Authority
1050 US 127 South
West Frankfort Office
   Complex
Frankfort, KY 40601

Louisiana
504-922-1038
Governor's Special
   Commission on
   Education Services
PO Box 91202
Baton Rouge, LA
   70821-9202

Maine
207-289-2183
Division of Higher
   Education Services
Department of
   Education and
   Cultural Services
Augusta, ME 04333

Maryland
301-333-6420
State Scholarship
   Board
2100 Guilford Avenue,
   Room 207
Baltimore, MD 21218

Massachusetts
617-727-9420
Board of Regents of
   Higher Education
Scholarship Office
330 Stuart Street
Boston, MA 02116

Michigan
517-373-3394
Michigan Higher
   Education
   Assistance
   Authority
PO Box 30008
Lansing, MI 48909

Minnesota
612-296-3974
Minnesota Higher
   Education
   Coordinating Board
Capitol Square
   Building, #400
550 Cedar Street
St. Paul, MN 55101

Mississippi
601-982-6570
Board of Trustees of
   State Institutions of
   Higher Learning
Student Financial Aid
PO Box 2336
Jackson, MS
   39225-2336

Missouri
314-751-3940
Coordinating Board
   for Higher
   Education
PO Box 1438
Jefferson City, MO
   65102

Montana
406-444-6594
Commission of Higher
   Education
35 South Last Chance
   Gulch
Helena, MT 59620

Nebraska
402-471-2847
Nebraska
   Coordinating
   Commission for
   Postsecondary
   Education
State Capitol
   Building, Sixth
   Floor
Lincoln, NE 68509

Nevada
702-784-4666
Financial Aid Office
U. of Nevada, Reno,
   Room 300 TSSC
Reno, NV 89557

New Hampshire
603-271-2555
New Hampshire
   Postsecondary
   Education
   Commission
2½ Beacon Street
Concord, NH 03301

New Jersey
609-588-3272,
800-792-8670
Department of Higher
   Education
Office of Student
   Assistance
4 Quakerbridge Plaza,
   CN 540
Trenton, NJ 08625

New Mexico
505-827-8300
Commission on
   Higher Education
1068 Cerrillos Road
Santa Fe, NM 87503

New York
518-474-5642
Higher Education
 Services
 Commission
99 Washington
 Avenue
Albany, NY 12255

North Carolina
919-549-8614
State Education
 Assistance
 Authority
Box 2688
Chapel Hill, NC 27515

North Dakota
701-224-4114
Student Financial
 Assistance Program
Capitol Building, 10th
 Floor
Bismark, ND 58505

Ohio
614-466-7420
Ohio Board of
 Regents
30 East Broad Street,
 36th Floor
Columbus, OH
 43266-0217

Oklahoma
405-521-2444
Oklahoma State
 Regents for Higher
 Education
500 Education
 Building
State Capitol Complex
Oklahoma City, OK
 73105

Oregon
503-686-4166
State Scholarship
 Commission
1445 Willamette
 Street, #9
Eugene, OR 97401

Pennsylvania
717-257-2800, (PA)
800-692-7435
Higher Education
 Assistance
 Authority
Town House, 660 Boas
 Street
Harrisburg, PA 17102

Rhode Island
401-277-2050
Higher Education
 Assistance
 Authority
560 Jefferson
 Boulevard
Warwick, RI 02886

South Carolina
803-734-1200
South Carolina Tuition
 Grants Agency
PO Box 12159, 411
 Keenan Building
Columbia, SC 29211

South Dakota
605-773-3134
Office of the Secretary
Department of
 Education and
 Cultural Affairs
700 Governors Drive
Pierre, SD 57501-2291

Tennessee
615-741-1346,
800-342-1663
Tennessee Student
 Assistance
 Corporation
404 James Robertson
 Parkway
Parkway Towers,
 Suite 1950
Nashville, TN 37219

Texas
512-462-6325
Texas Higher
 Education
 Coordinating Board
Box 12788, Capitol
 Station
Austin, TX 78711

Utah
801-538-5247
Utah State Board of
 Regents
335 W.N. Temple, 3
 Triad, Suite 550
Salt Lake City, UT
 84180-1205

Vermont
802-655-9602
Vermont Student
 Assistance
 Corporation
Champlain Mill, Box
 2000
Winooski, VT 05404

Virginia
804-225-2141
Council of Higher
 Education
James Monroe
 Building
101 North 14th Street
Richmond, VA 23219

Washington
206-753-3571
Higher Education
 Coordinating Board
917 Lake Ridge Way,
 GV-11
Olympia, WA 98504

West Virginia
304-347-1211
Higher Education
 Grant Program
PO Box 4007
Charleston, WV 25364

Wisconsin
608-266-2578
State of Wisconsin
 Higher Education
 Aids Board
PO Box 7885
Madison, WI 53707

Wyoming
307-766-2116
University of
Wyoming
Student Financial
Aids
Box 3335, University
Station
Laramie, WY 82071

Guam
617-734-2921, x3657
Financial Aid Office
University of Guam
UOG Station
Mangilao, GU 96923

Puerto Rico
809-758-3550
Council on Higher
Education
Box 23305, UPR
Station
Rio Piedras, PR 00931

Virgin Islands
809-774-4546
Board of Education
Commandant Gade,
OV #11
St. Thomas, VI 00801

For armed forces scholarships, contact your local recruiter.

Other scholarships and loans may be available through the following organizations:

The Federal Student Aid Information Center
PO Box 84
Washington, DC 20044

The Foundation of the National Student Nurses' Association, Inc.
555 West 57th Street
New York, NY 10019

Health Professional Scholarship Program (143B)
Veterans Affairs
Central Office
810 Vermont Avenue, NW
Washington, DC 20420

NHSC Scholarship Program
5600 Fishers Lane
Rockville, MD 20857

Nursing Education Assured Access Program
American Association of Colleges of Nursing
One Dupont Circle
Washington, DC 20036

U.S. Office of Education
Bureau of Student Financial Assistance
400 Maryland Avenue, SW
Washington, DC 20024

U.S. Public Health Service
Bureau of Health Manpower, Student Assistance Branch
5600 Fishers Lane
Rockville, MD 20857

United Student Aid Funds
8115 Knue Road
Indianapolis, IN 46250

Questions and Answers on The Computerized NCLEX-RN Exam

ALICE M. STEIN AND BARBARA T. LICHT

1. **WHAT IS THE NEW COMPUTERIZED NATIONAL COUNCIL LICENSING EXAMINATION (NCLEX-RN)?**

   It is a new way of administering the RN licensure examination. Rather than the traditional paper-and-pencil format, the examination utilizes computer technology.

   The basic exam remains the same. That is, the test still consists of a series of multiple choice questions. Like all exams, you are never tested on everything in a subject area—you are just tested on a representative sample. The computerized exam uses the same principle—it measures a sample of the subject area—however, it does this in a new way. It custom tailors a test for each candidate. The computer adapts questions for each candidate based on the candidate's answer to the previous question. This is why it is called "Computerized Adaptive Testing" or "CAT."

2. **HOW DOES CAT DESIGN A CANDIDATE'S TEST?**

   There is a large pool of questions from which individual questions are pulled for each test. All the questions conform to a test plan sometimes known as the blueprint. Additionally, each question has a difficulty rating.

   The computer custom tailors an exam for a candidate using the following technique. The candidate is given a

Stein, Alice M. and Licht, Barbara T., "Questions and Answers on the Computerized NCLEX-RN Exam." *Imprint Career Planning Guide 1994*, Vol. 41: No. 1, January, 1994, pp. 9–11. reprinted by permission, Medical College of Pennsylvania and the National Student Nurses' Association, Inc., New York, NY.

question. If they get it right, the next question will be
slightly more difficult. If they get it wrong, the next
question will be slightly easier. Every time they answer correctly, the next question will be a little more
difficult. And each time they answer incorrectly, the
next question will be slightly easier. Eventually, the
computer will determine the candidate's skill level.

3. DO I NEED TO BE FAMILIAR WITH COMPUTERS IN OR-
DER TO DO WELL ON THE NCLEX-RN?

No, you don't need to know anything at all about using computers in order to do well on the exam. In fact,
in a large trial, there was no significant difference between candidates experienced with computers and
those with no experience.

4. SHOULD I STUDY ANY DIFFERENTLY FOR THE COM-
PUTERIZED VERSION OF THE NCLEX-RN?

No. You will be tested on the same body of knowledge. All questions are still multiple choice, and the
only difference to the tester is that you are answering
the questions on the computer rather than using paper-
and-pencil. Like any major exam, you should be well
prepared before you take the test, ready to answer
questions on all aspects of nursing.

5. HOW MANY QUESTIONS ARE ON THE NCLEX-RN?

There is no set number of questions. The number will
vary with each candidate. The computer will end the
test when it has determined the candidate's skill level.

6. DOES THE EXAM HAVE A MINIMUM/MAXIMUM NUM-
BER OF QUESTIONS?

Yes. Each exam must contain at least 75 questions
and no more than 265.

7. ARE THERE ANY EXPERIMENTAL QUESTIONS?

Yes, there are at least 15 experimental questions on
each candidate's exam. You will have no way of knowing which ones they are and they do not count for or
against your score.

8. IS THERE A TIME LIMIT ON THE NCLEX-RN?

Candidates can take the amount of time they need—
up to a total of five hours. Most candidates will complete the exam in less than five hours.

9. WILL THERE BE LINKED QUESTIONS? THAT IS, WILL ONE QUESTION BE DEPENDENT ON ANOTHER?

No. Because of the nature of CAT, questions are not linked in any way. Remember, whether or not you get a question right determines what question will appear next. The questions on an exam cannot appear in any pre-set order.

10. CAN I SKIP A QUESTION?

No! Each question must be answered and you cannot go back to review a question or change your answer.

11. HOW DO I SIGN UP FOR THE NCLEX-RN?

You arrange to take the NCLEX-RN by applying to your state board of nursing for licensure as a registered nurse. Once your application is complete, your board of nursing will send you information. Included will be your candidate number. You will then call an 800 number to arrange your testing date. First-time examinees must be given an exam date that is within thirty days of their call.

12. WHERE DO I TAKE THE NCLEX-RN?

ETS and Sylvan/KEE Systems have a corporate partnership to administer the CAT NCLEX-RN. Sylvan/KEE systems has about 200 testing centers throughout the country. You pick the one you wish to use. Most likely, there will be one near you.

13. WHAT DOES A TESTING CENTER LOOK LIKE?

Testing centers are usually located in commercial buildings or shopping areas. They are modern and comfortable facilities run by the Sylvan/KEE systems. There is a registration area and a testing area. Each testing station contains a computer, is well lit, and is separated from other test stations by partitions.

14. HOW MANY CANDIDATES MAY TAKE THE EXAM AT ONE TIME?

The testing sites have up to ten computers—so up to ten candidates can take the exam at any one time.

15. I UNDERSTAND THAT I WILL BE ASKED TO SIGN A CONFIDENTIALITY STATEMENT. WHAT IS THE PURPOSE OF THIS?

Since candidates will take the exam at different times, it is vital that the integrity of the test questions be maintained. This is an important legal and ethical issue. **It is crucial that you not share any information about the test items with anyone.** In order to ensure confidentiality, the National Council requires all candidates to sign a nondisclosure statement prior to taking the exam.

16. WILL I BE ABLE TO PRACTICE ON THE COMPUTER BEFORE I TAKE THE NCLEX-RN?

Yes. On the day of your exam, prior to starting the actual test, you will be given a computer tutorial. This will familiarize you with how the computer works and gives you an opportunity to practice before you begin the exam.

17. WILL THERE BE ANY REST BREAKS DURING THE EXAM?

Yes. There is a mandatory ten-minute break after two testing hours. There is an optional break after an additional one and one-half hours. The short tutorial and all rest breaks are counted as part of the five-hour maximum test time.

18. WHAT SHOULD I WEAR WHEN I TAKE THE EXAM?

Wear comfortable clothes on the day of the exam. Also, be prepared by wearing layers of clothing so that you are not too warm or too cold. It is important that you be comfortable so that you can put all your energy into answering the questions!

19. HOW OFTEN WILL THE NCLEX-RN BE GIVEN?

Testing will be available year-round, 15 hours per day, 6 days per week, and on Sundays when necessary.

20. WHEN WILL I KNOW THE RESULTS?

Your state board of nursing will mail you the results. The amount of time from when you take the exam until you receive your results will vary from state to state. However, under the new system you should receive notification much faster.

21. IF I DON'T PASS, HOW SOON CAN I RETAKE THE NCLEX-RN?

Candidates who fail the exam can retest in three months.

U.S. State and Territorial Boards of Nursing

Alabama
Board of Nursing
RSA Plaza, Suite 250
770 Washington
  Avenue
Montgomery, AL
  36130-3900

Alaska
Board of Nursing
  Licensing
Department of
  Commerce and
  Economic
  Development
Division of
  Occupational
  Licensing
PO Box 110806
Juneau, AK
  99811-0806

Arizona
Board of Nursing
2001 West Camelback
  Road, Suite 350
Phoenix, AZ 85015

Arkansas
Board of Nursing
University Tower
  Building, Suite 800
1123 South University
  Avenue
Little Rock, AR 72204

California
Board of Registered
  Nursing
PO Box 944210
  400 R Street, Suite
  4030
Sacramento, CA 95814

Colorado
Board of Nursing
1560 Broadway, Suite
  670
Denver, CO 80202

Connecticut
Board of Examiners
  for Nursing
150 Washington
  Street
Hartford, CT 06106

Delaware
Board of Nursing
Margaret O'Neill
  Building
PO Box 1401
Federal and Court
  Streets
Dover, DE 19903

District of Columbia
Board of Nursing
614 H Street NW,
  Room 904
Washington, DC 20001

Florida
Board of Nursing
111 East Coastline
  Drive, Suite 504
Jacksonville, FL
  32202

Georgia
Board of Nursing
166 Pryor Street SW,
  Suite 400
Atlanta, GA 30303

Guam
Board of Nurse
  Examiners
Box 2816
Agana, GU 96910

Hawaii
Board of Nursing
Box 3469
Honolulu, HI 96801

Idaho
Board of Nursing
280 North Eighth
  Street, Suite 210
Boise, ID 83720

Illinois
Department of
  Professional
  Regulation
320 West Washington
  Street, Third Floor
Springfield, IL 62786

Indiana
Indiana State Board
  of Nursing
Health Professions
  Bureau
402 West Washington
  Street, Room 041
Indianapolis, IN 46204

Iowa
Board of Nursing
1223 East Court
Des Moines, IA 50319

Kansas
Board of Nursing
Landon State Office
  Building
900 SW Jackson, Suite
  551
Topeka, KS
  66612-1230

Kentucky
Board of Nursing
312 Whittington
  Parkway, Suite 300
Louisville, KY
  40222-5172

Louisiana
Board of Nursing
150 Baronne Street,
  Room 912
New Orleans, LA
  70112

Maine
Board of Nursing
State House
  Station 158
Augusta, ME 04333

Maryland
Board of Nursing
Metro Executive
  Center
4201 Patterson
  Avenue
Baltimore, MD
  21215-2299

Massachusetts
Board of Registration
  in Nursing
100 Cambridge Street,
  Room 1519
Boston, MA 02202

Michigan
Board of Nursing
PO Box 30018
Lansing, MI 48909

Minnesota
Board of Nursing
2700 University
  Avenue W, #108
St. Paul, MN 55114

Mississippi
Board of Nursing
239 North Lamar
  Street, Suite 401
Jackson, MS
  39201-1311

Missouri
Board of Nursing
PO Box 656
Jefferson City, MO
  65102

Montana
Board of Nursing
Department of
  Commerce
Arcade Building,
  Lower Level
111 North Jackson
PO Box 200513
Helena, MT
  59620-0513

Nebraska
Board of Nursing
PO Box 95007
Lincoln, NE 68509

Nevada
Board of Nursing
1281 Terminal Way,
  Suite 116
Reno, NV 89502

New Hampshire
Board of Nursing
Division of Public
  Health Service
Health and Welfare
  Building
6 Hazen Drive
Concord, NH
  03301-6527

New Jersey
Board of Nursing
124 Halsey Street,
  Sixth Floor
PO Box 45010
Newark, NJ 07101

New Mexico
Board of Nursing
4253 Montgomery
  Boulevard, NE,
  Suite 130
Albuquerque, NM
  87109

New York
Board of Nursing
State Education
  Department
Cultural Education
  Center, Room 3013
Albany, NY 12230

North Carolina
Board of Nursing
PO Box 2189
Raleigh, NC 27602

North Dakota
Board of Nursing
919 South Seventh
  Street, Suite 504
Bismarck, ND
  58504-5881

Ohio
Board of Nursing
77 South High Street,
  17th Floor
Columbus, OH
  43266-0316

Oklahoma
Board of Nurse
  Registration and
  Nursing Education
2915 North Classen
  Boulevard, Suite
  524
Oklahoma City, OK
  73106

Oregon
Board of Nursing
800 NE Oregon
  Street, Suite #25465
Portland, OR 97232

Pennsylvania
Board of Nursing
PO Box 2649
Harrisburg, PA
  17105-2649

Puerto Rico
Puerto Rico Board of
  Nurse Examiners
Box 10200
Santurce, PR
  00908-0200

Rhode Island
Board of Nurse
  Registration and
  Nursing Education
Cannon Health
  Building, Room 104
3 Capitol Hill
Providence, RI
  02908-2488

South Carolina
Board of Nursing
220 Executive Center
  Drive, Suite 220
Columbia, SC 29210

South Dakota
Board of Nursing
3307 South Lincoln
  Avenue
Sioux Falls, SD
  57105-5224

Tennessee
Board of Nursing
Bureau of Manpower
  and Facilities
283 Plus Park
  Boulevard
Nashville, TN
  37247-1010

Texas
Board of Nurse
  Examiners
9101 Burnet Road,
  Suite 104
Austin, TX 78758

Utah
Division of
  Occupational and
  Professional
  Licensing
Board of Nursing
Heber M. Wells
  Building, Fourth
  Floor
160 East 300 South
PO Box 45805
Salt Lake City, UT
  84145

Vermont
Board of Nursing
109 State Street
Montpelier, VT
  05609-1106

Virgin Islands
Board of Nurse
  Licensure
Gov't Hill
Kongens Gade #3
St. Thomas, VI 00803

Virginia
Board of Nursing
6606 West Broad
  Street, Fourth
  Floor
Richmond, VA
  23230-1717

Washington
PO Box 47864
Olympia, WA
  98504-7864

West Virginia
Board of Examiners
  for Registered
  Nurses
101 Dee Drive
Charleston, WV
  25311-1620

Wisconsin
Board of Nursing
PO Box 8935
Madison, WI
  53708-8935

Wyoming
Board of Nursing
Barrett Building,
  Second Floor
2301 Central Avenue
Cheyenne, WY 82002

American Samoa
Health Service
  Regulatory Board
LBJ Tropical Medical
  Center
Pago Pago, American
  Samoa 96799

**Northern Mariana
  Islands**
Commonwealth Board
  of Nurse Examiners
Public Health Center
PO Box 1458
Saipan, MP 96950

U.S. and Canadian Nursing Organizations

UNITED STATES

American Nurses' Association
600 Maryland Avenue SW, Suite 100 West
Washington, DC 20024-2571

National League for Nursing
350 Hudson Street, Fourth Floor
New York, NY 10014

National Student Nurses' Association
555 West 57th Street
Room 1325
New York, NY 10019

State Associations

Alabama State Nurses
Association
360 North Hull Street
Montgomery, AL
36104-3658

Alaska Nurses
Association
237 East Third
Avenue
Anchorage, AK 99501

Arizona Nurses
Association
1850 East Southern
Avenue, Suite 1
Tempe, AZ 85282-5832

Arkansas State
Nurses Association
117 South Cedar
Little Rock, AR 72205

California Nurses
Association
1145 Market Street,
11th Floor
San Francisco, CA
94103

Colorado Nurses
Association
5453 East Evans
Place
Denver, CO 80222

Connecticut Nurses
Association
377 Research
Parkway, Suite 2D
Meriden, CT 06450

Delaware Nurses
Association
2634 Capitol Trail,
Suite A
Newark, DE 19711

District of Columbia
Nurses Association
5100 Wisconsin
Avenue NW, Suite
306
Washington, DC 20016

Florida Nurses
Association
1235 East Concord
Street
PO Box 536985
Orlando, FL
32853-6985

Georgia Nurses
Association
1362 West Peachtree
Street NW
Atlanta, GA 30309

Guam Nurses
Association
35 Rota Street
Santa Rita, GU 96915

Hawaii Nurses
Association
677 Ala Moana
Boulevard, Suite
301
Honolulu, HI 96813

Idaho Nurses
Association
200 North Fourth
Street, Suite 20
Boise, ID 83702-6001

Illinois Nurses
Association
300 South Wacker
Drive
Chicago, IL 60606

Indiana State Nurses
Association
2915 North High
School Road
Indianapolis, IN
46224-2969

Iowa Nurses
Association
One Corporate Place
1501 42nd Street,
Suite 471
West Des Moines, IA
50265

Kansas State Nurses
Association
700 SW Jackson, Suite
601
Topeka, KS
66603-3731

Kentucky Nurses
Association
PO Box 2616
1400 South First
Street
Louisville, KY 40201

Louisiana State
Nurses Association
712 Transcontinental
Drive
Metairie, LA 70001

Maine State Nurses
Association
295 Water Street
PO Box 2240
Augusta, ME
04330-2240

Maryland Nurses
Association
849 International
Drive
Airport Square XXI,
Suite 255
Linthicum, MD 21090

Massachusetts Nurses
Association
340 Turnpike Street
Canton, MA 02021

Michigan Nurses
Association
2310 Jolly Oak Road
Okemus, MI 48864

Minnesota Nurses
Association
1295 Bandana
Boulevard N, Suite
140
St. Paul, MN 55108

Mississippi Nurses
Association
135 Bounds Street
Jackson, MS 39206

Missouri Nurses
Association
206 East Dunklin
Street
PO Box 325
Jefferson City, MO
65102-0325

Montana Nurses
Association
PO Box 5718
Helena, MT 59604

Nebraska Nurses
Association
941 "O" Street, Suite
711
Lincoln, NE 68508

Nevada Nurses
Association
3660 Baker Lane,
Suite 104
Reno, NV 89509

New Hampshire
Nurses Association
48 West Street
Concord, NH 03301

New Jersey State
Nurses Association
320 West State Street
Trenton, NJ 08618

New Mexico Nurses
Association
909 Virginia, NE,
Suite 101
Albuquerque, NM
87108

New York State
Nurses Association
2113 Western Avenue
Guilderland, NY
12084

North Carolina
Nurses Association
Box 12025
Raleigh, NC
27605-2025

North Dakota State
Nurses Association
212 North Fourth
Street
Bismarck, ND 58501

Ohio Nurses
Association
4000 East Main Street
Columbus, OH
43213-2983

Oklahoma Nurses
Association
6414 North Santa Fe,
Suite A
Oklahoma City, OK
73116

Oregon Nurses
Association
9600 SW Oak Street,
Suite 550
Portland, OR 97223

Pennsylvania Nurses
Association
2578 Interstate Drive
PO Box 68525
Harrisburg, PA
17106-8525

Puerto Rico
Colegio de
Professionales de la
Enfermeria de
Puerto Rico
PO Box 363647
San Juan, PR
00936-3647

Rhode Island State
Nurses Association
300 Ray Drive, Suite 5
Providence, RI
02906-4887

South Carolina
Nurses Association
1821 Gadsden Street
Columbia, SC 29201

South Dakota Nurses
Association
1505 South Minnesota,
Suite 6
Sioux Falls, SD 57105

Tennessee Nurses
Association
545 Mainstream
Drive, Suite 405
Nashville, TN
37228-1207

Texas Nurses
Association
7600 Burner Road,
Suite 440
Austin, TX 78757-1292

Utah Nurses
Association
455 East 400 South,
#402
Salt Lake City, UT
84111

Vermont State Nurses
Association
500 Dorset Street
South Burlington, VT
05403

Virgin Island Nurses
Association
PO Box 2866
Veterans Drive
Station
St. Thomas, VI 00803

Virginia Nurses
Association
1311 High Point
Avenue
Richmond, VA 23230

Washington State
Nurses Association
2505 Second Avenue,
Suite 500
Seattle, WA 98121

West Virginia Nurses
Association
PO Box 1946
Charleston, WV 25237

Wisconsin Nurses
Association
6117 Monona Drive
Madison, WI 53716

Wyoming Nurses
Association
Majestic Building,
Room 305
1603 Capitol Avenue
Cheyenne, WY 82001

CANADA

CANADIAN NURSES' ASSOCIATION
50 The Driveway
Ottawa, Ontario, Canada K2P 1E2

Canadian Provincial Registered Nurses Associations

Alberta
Alberta Association of
Registered Nurses
11620 168th Street
Edmonton, Alberta
T5M 4A6

British Columbia
Registered Nurses
Association of
British Columbia
2855 Arbutus Street
Vancouver, British
Columbia V6J 3Y8

Manitoba
Manitoba Association
of Registered
Nurses
647 Broadway Avenue
Winnipeg, Manitoba
R3C 0X2

New Brunswick
Nurse Association of
New Brunswick
231 Saunders Street
Fredericton, New
Brunswick E3B 1N6

Newfoundland
Association of
Registered Nurses
of Newfoundland
ARRN House
55 Military Road
Box 6116
St. Johns,
Newfoundland
A1C 5X8

Northwest Territories
Northwest Territories Registered Nurses Association
PO Box 2757
Yellowknife, Northwest Territories
X0E 1H0

Nova Scotia
Registered Nurses Association of Nova Scotia
6035 Coburt Road
Halifax, Nova Scotia
B3H 1Y8

Ontario
Registered Nurses Association of Ontario
33 Print Street
Toronto, Ontario
M4W 1Z2

Prince Edward Island
Association of Nurses of Prince Edward Island
41 Palmers Lane
PO Box 1838
Charlottetown, Prince Edward Island
C1A 7N5

Quebec
Order of Nurses of the Province of Quebec
4200 Dorchester Boulevard West
Montreal, Quebec
H3Z 1V4

Saskatchewan
Saskatchewan Registered Nurses Association
2066 Retallack Street
Regina, Saskatchewan
S4T 2K2

Yukon
Yukon Nurses Society
Box 5371
Whitehorse, Yukon
Y1A 4Z2

Specialized Nursing Organizations in the United States and Canada

U.S. ORGANIZATIONS

American Academy of Ambulatory Nursing Administration
North Woodbury Road, Box 56
Pitman, NJ 08071

American Academy of Nurse Practitioners
Capitol Station
LBJ Building
PO Box 12846
Austin, TX 78711

The American Assembly for Men in Nursing
PO Box 31753
Independence, OH 44131

American Association of Colleges of Nursing
One Dupont Circle NW, Suite 530
Washington, DC 20036

American Association of Critical-Care Nurses
101 Columbia
Aliso Viejo, CA 92656-1491

American Association of Nephrology Nurses and Technicians
Suite 219
505 North Tustin
Santa Ana, Ca 92705

American Association of Neuroscience Nurses
224 N. Des Plaines
Suite 601
Chicago, IL 60661

American Association of Neurosurgical Nurses
Suite 1519
625 North Michigan Avenue
Chicago, IL 60611

American Association of Nurse Anesthetists
222 South Prospect Avenue
Park Ridge, IL 60068-4001

American Association of Nurse Attorneys (TAANA)
720 Light Street
Baltimore, MD 21230

American Association of Occupational Health Nurses, Inc.
50 Lenox Pointe
Atlanta, GA 30324

American Association of Office Nurses
109 Kinderkamack Road
Montvale, NJ 07645

American Association of Spinal Cord Injury Nurses
75-20 Astoria Boulevard
Jackson Heights, NY 11370-1177

American College of Nurse-Midwives
1522 K Street NW, Suite 1000
Washington, DC 20005

American Holistic Nurses' Association
4101 Lake Boone Trail, Suite 201
Raleigh, NC 27606

American Indian/Alaska Native Nurses Association, Inc.
PO Box 1588
Norman, OK 7307

American
Nephrology
Nurses'
Association
North Woodbury
Road, Box 56
Pitman, NJ 08071

American
Organization of
Nurse Executives
840 North Lake Shore
Drive
Chicago, IL 60611

American
Psychiatric
Nurses'
Association
6900 Grove Road
Thorofare, NJ 08086

American
Radiological
Nurses
Association
c/o Elaine Deutsch
Plankey
2462 Stantonsburg
Road, Suite 162
Greenville, NC 27834

American Society of
Ophthalmic
Registered
Nurses, Inc.
655 Beach Street
PO Box 193030
San Francisco, CA
94119

American Society of
Plastic and
Reconstructive
Surgical Nurses,
Inc.
North Woodbury
Road, Box 56
Pitman, NJ 08071

American Society of
Post Anesthesia
Nurses
11512 Allecingie
Parkway, Suite C
Richmond, VA 23235

Association of
Nurses in AIDS
Care
704 Stonyhill Road,
Suite 106
Yardley, PA 19067

Association of
Operating Room
Nurses
2170 South Parker
Road
Suite 300
Denver, CO
80231-5711

Association of
Pediatric
Oncology Nurses
11512 Allecingie
Parkway
Richmond, VA 23235

Association of
Rehabilitation
Nurses
5700 Old Orchard
Road, First Floor
Skokie, IL 60077

Association of
Women's Health,
Obstetric, and
Neonatal Nurses
(AWHONN)
1101 Connecticut
Avenue NW, Suite
400
Washington, DC 20036

Dermatology Nurses
Association
North Woodbury
Road, Box 56
Pitman, NJ 08071

Drug and Alcohol
Nursing
Association, Inc.
Box 92 Lonely
Cottage Drive
Upper Black Eddy,
PA 18972

Emergency Nurses
Association
216 Higgins Road
Park Ridge, IL 60068

Gay Nurses Alliance
PO Box 115
Brownsville, TX 78520

Hospice Nurses
Association
2941 Highridge Road
La Crescenta, CA
91214

Intravenous Nurses
Society, Inc.
Two Brighton Street
Belmont, MA 02178

The National
Alliance of Nurse
Practitioners
325 Pennsylvania
Avenue SE
Washington, DC
20003-1100

National Association
of Directors of
Nursing
Administration in
Long Term Care
10999 Reed Hartman
Highway, Suite 234
Cincinnati, OH 45242

National Association
of Hispanic
Nurses
1501 Sixteenth Street
NW
Washington, DC 20036

National Association
of Neonatal
Nurses
1304 Southpoint
Boulevard, Suite
280
Petaluma, CA
94954-6859

National Association
of Orthopaedic
Nurses, Inc.
North Woodbury
Road, Box 56
Pitman, NJ 08071

**National Association
of Pediatric Nurse
Associates and
Practitioners**
1101 Kings Highway,
Suite 206
Cherry Hill, NJ 08034

**National Association
of Physician
Nurses**
900 South Washington
Street, Suite G-13
Falls Church, VA
22046

**National Association
of School Nurses,
Inc.**
PO Box 1300
Lamplighter Lane
Scarborough, ME
04074-1300

**National Black
Nurses
Association, Inc.**
1012 Tenth Street NW
Washington, DC 20001

**National Consortium
of Chemical
Dependency
Nurses**
1720 Willow Creek
Circle, Suite 519
Eugene, OR 97402

**National Council of
State Boards of
Nursing, Inc.**
676 North St. Clair,
Suite 550
Chicago, IL
60611-2921

**National Flight
Nurses
Association**
6900 Grove Road
Thorofare, NJ 08086

**National Male
Nurses'
Association**
2308 State Street
Saginaw, MI 48602

**Nurses Christian
Fellowship**
6400 Schroeder Road
PO Box 7895
Madison, WI
53707-7895

**Nurse Consultants
Association, Inc.**
414 Plaza Drive, Suite
209
Westmont, IL 60559

**Nurses Educational
Funds, Inc.**
555 West 57th Street
New York, NY 10019

**Nurses
Environmental
Health Watch**
181 Marshall Street
Duxbury, MA 02143

Nurses House, Inc.
350 Hudson Street
New York, NY 10014

**Oncology Nursing
Society**
501 Holiday Drive
Pittsburgh, PA 15220

**Public Health
Nursing/American
Public Health
Association**
1015 Fifteenth Street
NW
Washington, DC 20005

Sigma Theta Tau
International Honor
Society of Nursing
1100 Waterway
Boulevard
Indianapolis, IN 46202

**Society of
Gastroenterology
Nurses and
Associates, Inc.**
1070 Sibley Tower
Rochester, NY 14604

**The Society for
Nursing History**
Nursing Education
Department
Box 150
Teachers College
Columbia University
New York, NY 10027

**Society of
Otorhinolaryngo-
logy and
Head/Neck
Nurses**
116 Canal Street,
Suite A
New Smyrna Beach,
FL 32168

**Society for
Peripheral
Vascular Nursing**
309 Winter Street
Norwood, MA 02062

**Society of
Respiratory
Nursing**
5700 Old Orchard
Road, First Floor
Skokie, IL 60077-1024

**Transcultural
Nursing Society**
College of Nursing
and Health
Madonna University
36600 Schoolcraft
Road
Livonia, MI 48150

CANADIAN ORGANIZATIONS

Canadian Association of Critical Care Nurses
PO Box 61
Welland, Ontario
L3B 5N9

Canadian Association of Neurological and Neurosurgical Nurses
296 Palace Road
Kingston, Ontario
17L 4T3

Canadian Association of Practical and Nursing Assistants
RR #4
St. Stephen, New Brunswick
E3L 2Y2

Canadian Association of University Schools of Nursing
1200-151 Slater
Ottawa, Ontario
K1P 5N1

Canadian Council of Cardiovascular Nurses
1200-1 Nicholas Street
Ottawa, Ontario
K1N 7B7

Canadian Intravenous Nurses Association
200-4433 Sheppard Avenue E
Agincourt, Ontario
M1S 1V3

Canadian Orthopedic Nurses Association
43 Wellesley Street E
Toronto, Ontario
M4Y 1H1

Canadian University Nursing Students Association
School of Nursing
Universite de Montreal
C.P. 6128
Montreal, Quebec
H3T 1J4

Operating Room Nurses Association of Canada
213-52377 Range Road
Sherwood Park, Alberta T8G 1B9

Psychiatric Nurses Association of Canada
1854 Portage Avenue
Winnipeg, Manitoba
R3J 0G9

TPN Nurses Association of Canada
PO Box 62
Station K
Toronto, Ontario
M4P 2G1

Index

A

Ability, lack of, 86–87
Absenteeism, 87
Activities, outside, 88
American Hospital Association Bill of Rights, 145–147
American Nurses' Association Code for Nurses, 148–149
Anxiety
  with nursing skills lab, 141–142
  test, 76
Assertive nursing students, 61–62
Assertiveness, 62–63
Associate degree nursing program, 17–21
Attendance, class, 45
Attitudes
  judgmental, 114–115
  of nursing students, 39

B

Baccalaureate nursing program, 17–21
Behaviors, self-defeating, 87
Bill of Rights
  American Hospital Association, 145–148
  patients', 145–148
Bill of Rights and Responsibilities, Student, 152–154
Boards of Nursing, U.S. State and Territorial, 197–199
Budgeting of time, 45–46
Busywork, 49

C

Canadian Boards of Nursing, 197–199
Canadian nursing organizations, 203–204
   specialized, 208
Canadian University Nursing Students' Association, 102
Career, selection of, 5–6
Children, support from, 131–132
Class attendance, 45
Class time, utilizing, 67–69
Clinical component, 139–143
   instructors and, 159–160
Code for Nurses, American Nurses' Association, 148–149
Commitment, lack of, 86
Communication, nonverbal, 162–163
Concentrating, 46
Consent, informed, 152, 154–156
Contingency plans, 134
Copies, 51
Costs of nursing education, 23–27

D

Decision making, 51, 125
Detours, 53–57
Diploma nursing program, 17–21
Dirty jobs, 46
Dress codes, 30–31

E

Education, nursing, costs of, 23–27
Effectiveness, increasing, 43–51
Efficiency, increasing, 43–51
80/20 principle, 44–45
Electives, 109–111
Equipment, 46–47
Essay test questions, tips for, 81–82
Exams, questions and answers, 193–196
Exams, state board, 83; *see also* Tests

F

Failures, 85–89
Family support, 129–132
Filing system, 47

Fill-in-the-blank questions, tips for, 80
Financial aid, 24–26

G

Goals, 47–48, 54–57
Grades and mature students, 134–136
Graduation, preparation for, 165–167
Grants, 24
Grievance procedure guidelines, 177–181
Group support, 97–98
Guessing on test, 82
Guilt, 50
Guilt trips, 6

H

Habits, study, poor, 87–88
Health professions, women in, ten basic rights for, 151
Help, asking for, 59–63
Homesickness, 97–98
Hospital, clinical work in, 139–143, 159–163
Housekeeping help, 129–130

I

Illness, 86
Informed consent, 152, 154–156
Instructors, 37–41
    and clinical practice, 159–160
    degrees needed for, 39–40
    responsibilities of, 40–41
    and tests, 76–77
Insurance, malpractice, 155–156

J

Jobs, part-time, for nursing students, 57
Journal, keeping, 106–107
Judgmental attitudes, 114–115

L

Lawsuits, 154–155
Laziness, 86
Legal implications for nursing, 154–156

Librarian, 49
Library, reference, personal, 46–47
Lifestyle, 105–107
Lists, 48–49
Loans, sources of, 189–191
Long-term memory, 69–73

M

Malpractice insurance, 155–156
Mandatory overtime, 14
Married students, 129–132; *See also* Mature students
Matching questions, tips for, 80
Mathematical tests questions, tips for, 80–81
Mature students, 127–137
    family support for, 129–132
    grades and, 135–136
    personal vs professional lives for, 135–136
    shifting gears by, 136–137
Memory, 65–73
    improving, 66–67
    reading to increase, 69–73
    short-term, 65
Men in nursing, 134
Mnemonics to increase memory, 67
Multiple-choice questions, tips for 79

N

National Student Nurses' Association, 102
    grievance procedure guidelines of, 177–181
Networking, 100–101
Nonverbal communication, 162–163
Notes
    class, 68–69
    on reading, 71
    reviewing, 69–70
Notetaking, abbreviations for, 68–69
Nurses
    Code for, American Nurses' Association, 148–149
    demand for, 6–7
    duties of, 7–8
    qualities needed in, 8–9
    salaries for, 12–15

shortage of, effects of, 13–14
skills of, keeping current, 7–8
Nursing
alternative in, 113–115
as career, selections of, 5–6
job security in, 6
legal implications for, 154–156
men in, 134
role of, in patient rights, 149–151
Nursing education, costs of, 23–27
Nursing organizations, U.S. and Canadian, 201–204
specialized, 205–207
Nursing programs, comparison of, 17–21
Nursing school
finishing up, 165–167
rules of, 29–31
Nursing skills lab, 139–143
Nursing students
attitudes of, 39
group support for, 97–102
lifestyle of, 105–107
mature, 127–137; *see also* Mature students
part-time jobs for, 57
tips for, 33
Nursing texts, 70; *see also* Textbooks

O

Oral presentations, 117–121
rehearsal for, 118–121
Outside activities, 88
Overtime, mandatory, 14

P

Papers, 121–123
Parkinson's Law, 39
Part-time jobs for nursing students, 57
Passive nursing students, 61–63
Patients
beginning work with, 160
bills of rights for, 145–148
right of, role of nursing in, 149–152
Perfectionism, 49

Persistence, 59–61
Personal vs professional life, 135–136
Photocopying, 51
Positive attitudes, 39
Prefixes used in nursing, 183–187
Presentations, oral, 117–121
Prime time, 50
Priorities, 54–57
    setting, 44–45, 48–50
Procrastination, 50
    overcoming, 91–94
    psychology of, 92–93
Professional vs personal life, 135–136

Q

Questions, 50

R

Reading and remembering, 69–72
Reading skills, 70–72
Reference library, personal, 47
Regrets, 50
Resources, 173–175
Responsibility, 125
Reward system, 93–94
Rights
    of patients, role of nursing in, 149–152
    student, 151–156
        grievance procedure guidelines on, 177–181

S

Salaries of nurses, 12–15
Scholarships, 24
    sources of, 189–191
Self-defeating behaviors, 87
Self-pity, 50
Sequencing, 133
Short answer questions, tips for, 80
Short-term memory, 65
Sleep, 51
State board exams, 83
Student aid, 24–26

Student Bill of Rights and Responsibilities, 152–154
Student rights, 151–156
Students, nursing; *see* Nursing students
Study groups, 98–102
    improving, 100–101
Study habits, poor, 87
Suffixes used in nursing, 187
Support groups, 99, 100–102
    advantages of, 98–99
Survival tips, 33–35

T

Teachers, 37–41
    and clinical practice, 159–160
    degrees needed for, 40
    responsibilities of, 40–41
    and tests, 76–77
Teaching teams, 38–39
"Ten Basic Rights for Women in the Health Professions," 151
Tests, 75–76
    anxiety about, 75–76
    guessing on, 82
    instructions for, 78
    preparation for, 76–83
    questions on, tips for answering, 79–82
    teacher and, 76–77
Textbooks
    cost of, 23
    purchasing, 46–47
    reading, 69–72
Time
    management of, 45–46, 50, 51
    others', planning for, 49–50
    prime, 50
    saving, 50
True-false questions, tips for, 79–80

U

U.S. nursing organizations, 201–204
    specialized, 205–208
U.S. State Boards of Nursing, 197–199

V

Visualization to increase memory, 66–67

W

Walk-on-Water Women, 133–134
"Women in the Health Professions, Ten Basic Rights for," 151